OXFORD MEDICAL PUBLICATIONS

Psychopharmacology of old age

BRITISH ASSOCIATION FOR PSYCHOPHARMACOLOGY MONOGRAPHS

1. Psychopharmacology of affective disorders
    edited by E. S. Paykel and A. Coppen

2. Psychopharmacology of anticonvulsants
    edited by Merton Sandler

3. Psychopharmacology of old age
    edited by David Wheatley

Psychopharmacology of old age

BRITISH ASSOCIATION
FOR PSYCHOPHARMACOLOGY
MONOGRAPH
No. 3

EDITED BY
DAVID WHEATLEY

Programme Secretary,
British Association for Psychopharmacology

OXFORD
OXFORD UNIVERSITY PRESS
NEW YORK TORONTO

Oxford University Press, Walton Street, Oxford OX2 6DP

London Glasgow New York Toronto
Delhi Bombay Calcutta Madras Karachi
Kuala Lumpur Singapore Hong Kong Tokyo
Nairobi Dar es Salaam Cape Town
Melbourne Auckland

and associate companies in
Beirut Berlin Ibadan Mexico City Nicosia
OXFORD is a trade mark of Oxford University Press

First published 1982
Reprinted and issued as a paperback 1983

British Library Cataloguing in Publication Data
Psychopharmacology of old age. — (Oxford Medical
publications). — (British Association for
Psychopharmacology Monograph; no. 3)
1. Geriatric psychopharmacology
2. Geriatrics — Congresses
I. Wheatley, David, 1919-   II. Series
618.97'68918   RC451.4
ISBN 0-19-261456-8

Library of Congress Cataloging in Publication Data
Main entry under title:
Psychopharmacology of old age.
    (British Association for Psychopharmacology
monograph; no. 3) (Oxford medical publications)
    Based upon the proceedings of a symposium held
in 1981 which was organized by the British Association
for Psychopharmacology
    Bibliography: p.
    Includes index.
    1. Geriatric pharmacology.   2. Psychopharmacology.
I. Wheatley, David, 1919-   II. British Association
for Psychopharmacology.   III. Series.
IV. Series: Oxford medical publications. [DNLM:
1. Psychopharmacology—In old age—Congresses.
2. Mental disorder—In old age—Congresses.
3. Cognition disorders—In old age—Congresses.
WM402 P9756 1981]
RC953.7.P78 1982   618.97 689061   82-8089
ISBN 0 – 19-261456-8   AACR2

Printed in Great Britain by
The Thetford Press Ltd, Thetford, Norfolk

Preface

The autumn of life should no longer be a period of forgotten dreams and unfulfilled endeavours, but rather one of emotional and mental fulfilment, now that advances in medical science have made it possible to halt or allay many of the physical ravages of age. But despite this, it may still be followed by a 'winter of discontent', in which disabilities of the mind are heavily implicated.

This volume is based upon the proceedings of a symposium of the same name, organized by the British Association for Psychopharmacology which, appropriately, took place in the autumn of 1981. As is the custom of the Association, the symposium embraced advances in both basic scientific and clinical areas, that have enhanced our knowledge and understanding of the aging process as it affects the mind, and the pharmacological means by which disorders of the same may be combated. The volume is divided into three sections, namely: Basic Concepts, Cognitive Disorders, and Psychiatric Disorders.

No one system or part of the body can be divorced from the organism as a whole and yet, when considering the elderly, that is what tends to happen. The physician treating his aged confused patient with pneumonia, is pleasantly surprised when the resolution of the bacterial infection is accompanied by a return to sanity. And yet there are many more subtle occasions when the physical component of psychomental changes in the old may be overlooked, just as the effects of the mind on the functioning of the body may be dismissed by the physician practising general medicine.

It is therefore appropriate that the first section of the book is concerned with, in the first instance, the nature of aging processes per se, this being followed by chapters on: experimental work in animals that may throw light on derangement of the thinking processes; the social implications of mental senility; the changes that age produces on drug action in the body; and the problems of ensuring adequate pharmacotherapy in the face of failing memory and cognition. Thus, the section on basic concepts spans present-day knowledge of the aging processes generally, from the cellular level, by way of experimental work that may hold hope for future treatment, to the practical problem of using the drugs at present available to their best advantage in elderly patients.

The second section of the book is concerned specifically with cognitive disorders of old age, and opens appropriately with two chapters on the isolation of a peptide that may have psychotropic and nootropic properties. Consequent upon these, intriguing possibilities arise for the understanding of the aging process. The brain possesses specific opiate and benzodiazepine receptors; the implication of which must be that either the body possesses also the appropriate ligands, or that nature's intent is for man to discover appropriate chemical compounds to bind to these receptors. Is it any more fanciful that the brain may also possess specific 'old age' receptors, that merely await our ingenuity in discovering the appropriate synthetic ligands?

But, to return to the present. Not too many drugs are available to treat the waning mental powers of old age and, 'improvement' being a relative state in the old, their effectiveness is difficult to determine. Thus, the therapeutic action of a nootropic drug may be manifested by prevention of further deterioration, rather than by actual improvement. Furthermore, a relatively small improvement that might pass undetected by recognized assessment measures, may produce profound effects on wellbeing in the old. Two chapters in this section are therefore concerned with the methods of measuring such subtle changes in the elderly, and assessing the effects of two of the relatively few drugs that are available to the clinician for treatment.

One of the most distressing facets of advancing years is the gradual, but inexorable, isolation of the elderly person from his social milieu. A harmonious relationship between an elderly relative and younger members of the family, is rendered more difficult by the restrictions imposed by financial problems and limited living-space; aspects of modern life that affect most of the community in one way or another. No longer is the grandparent an honoured guest in the house, waited on hand and foot, in return for the many years that he or she gave in service to the children. Differences in outlook, the changed role of younger women in the community, the ubiquitous quest for material advantages, are some of the factors that tend to create a situation that may become strained in the extreme. And so, increasingly the old are isolated from their kith and kin, whilst their equally elderly friends die off around them, and they become cut off from contact with others through their failing senses. And of these failing senses, impairment of hearing and eyesight are perhaps the most important, isolating the sufferer even from contact with the outside world through the media. No wonder that depression may be associated with such a state of affairs and this is considered in the concluding chapter of this section.

The harmonious use of the English language is not, perhaps, a usual feature of scientific work but, when combined with logical argument as in the chapter on anxiety in old age, it constitutes a formidable component in the section on psychiatric disorders. How many old people are prescribed more and more drugs, mainly of a symptomatic nature and sometimes just to 'keep them quiet'? Psychotropic drugs that are specifically potent in the young may merely worsen confusion and anxiety in the elderly. For any reader who is a firm advocate of psychopharmacology in old age, this chapter should signal the tempering of enthusiasm with sober reflection.

Depression on the other hand is a definitive illness and needs to be treated in the elderly just as much as in the young. Whilst the general principles are similar, due regard must be paid to the altered pharmacokinetics and, indeed, different symptom profiles that may require alternative choices for drug therapy. A further chapter in the book is devoted to these aspects of affective disorder in the geriatric community. Very similar considerations apply to the diagnosis and treatment of psychotic disorders and these are also considered in a separate chapter. For paraphrenia, as for depression, psychopharmacology must provide the prime means of successful treatment.

In the final chapter of the book, perhaps one of the most important aspects of psychopharmacology in old age is reviewed. It is agreed that reduced duration of sleep is a natural physiological process, as age increases into the fifth and sixth decades and beyond, but this is seldom appreciated by those who experience it. The psychological effects can be profound and should be taken into consideration when deciding whether or not to prescribe a hypnotic drug. There is no worse situation for the octogenarian widow or widower, retiring night after night, probably at an early hour as an escape from the boredom of sitting alone in a silent empty room, to awaken prematurely in the middle of the night when the safety of sleep was anticipated until the light of dawn. As with a child, so at night all things become magnified — the creak of the floorboards that might signal an intruder, the ticking of the clock that seems supernaturally loud, the squeaks and creaks of the building as it adapts to the colder night air that may signify the advent of marauding rodents, a displaced hair on the face felt as some obnoxious insect — and so on and so forth. No wonder that elderly people frequently turn on the lights during the night and, far from feeling refreshed from their short physiological sleep the next morning, spend a restless day worrying about what is going to happen on the next night, and the next night, and the next night after that. This may explain the predilection of many elderly patients for the longer-acting sleeping drugs, although of course physiologically these must be regarded as bad for them. And perhaps we should pause awhile to consider to what extent the clinician is justified in withholding such 'comfort drugs' from his patients.

This volume is therefore concerned with both the autumn and winter of life, and it is in the former period that psychopharmacology should find its most important application. Then, perhaps, we shall be able to prevent that most distressing spectacle of all — the patient who has been rendered old before a time to be old.

London   D. W.
February 1982

Contents

List of contributors

R. BRAITHWAITE,
Regional Toxicology Department,
Dudley Road Hospital,
Birmingham,
England

M. E. BRUCE,
ARC and MRC Neuropathogenesis Unit,
Edinburgh,
Scotland

A. COMFORT,
Neuropsychiatric Institute,
UCLA,
Los Angeles,
USA

P. CROME,
Department of Medicine for the Elderly,
St. Helen's Hospital,
Hastings,
Sussex,
England

A. J. CROSS,
Division of Psychiatry,
Clinical Research Centre,
Northwick Park Hospital,
Harrow,
England

T. J. CROW,
Division of Psychiatry,
Clinical Research Centre,
Northwick Park Hospital,
Harrow,
England

A. G. DICKINSON,
ARC and MRC Neuropathogenesis Unit,
Edinburgh,
Scotland

K. GILHOME HERBST,
The Mental Health Foundation,
London,
England

I. G. GROVE-WHITE,
Division of Psychiatry,
Clinical Research Centre,
Northwick Park Hospital,
Harrow,
England

D. E. HARRISON,
The Jackson Laboratory,
Bar Harbor,
Maine,
USA

D. JOLLEY,
Withington Hospital,
Manchester,
England

R. J. McDONALD,
Research Laboratories,
Schering AG,
Berlin,
West Germany

S. A. MONTGOMERY,
Academic Department of Psychiatry,
St. Mary's Hospital Medical School,
London,
England

P. W. OVERSTALL,
General Hospital,
Hereford,
England

R. M. PIGACHE,
Medical Unit,
Organon Scientific Development Group,
Oss,
The Netherlands

B. PITT,
The London Hospital,
London,
England

H. RIGTER,
Dutch Science Council,
The Hague,
The Netherlands

D. G. ROSS,
Division of Psychiatry,
Clinical Research Centre,
Northwick Park Hospital,
Harrow,
England

A. WHITEHEAD,
Department of Psychology,
Kingston and Richmond Area Health Authority, and
St. George's Hospital Medical School,
London,
England

PART I
Basic concepts

1

The nature of aging

DAVID E. HARRISON

To outline the nature of aging, I will begin by defining the aging process. This process causes an exponentially increasing risk of death from almost all causes throughout the adult lifetime. Creatures that age show an expontential increase in death risk with a linear increase in age, as illustrated in Fig. 1.1 (from Kohn 1978). The top line gives the death rate from all causes, and increases in a smooth exponential fashion between 30 and 80 years of age; and the next three lines show the increase with age in the risk of death from cardiovascular diseases, cancers, and two common types of infectious disease. All four show similar rates of increase, except that the rate of increase for death from cancer declines slightly after age 60. Such statistical information is discussed more thoroughly by Comfort (1979).

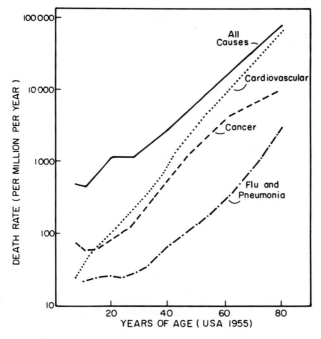

Fig. 1.1. This illustrates exponential increases in the total death rate from all causes and in death rates from cardiovascular diseases, cancers, or flu and pneumonia, with linear increases in age. (This figure uses data from Fig. 6.6 in Kohn (1978).)

AGING AND DEATH RATES

People generally define aging by what it does, because statistical information of the kind illustrated in Fig. 1.1 is reliable, repeatable, and easy to come by. Figure 1.2 illustrates how these curves would be changed by different processes. Line A in Fig. 1.2 shows the current rate of increase in death risk with increasing age. Line B in the same figure shows what would happen if 10 years was added to the lifespan. The rate of increase in death risk is unchanged, but the risk at any age would be the same as at a 10 year younger age in curve A. This is what happens in the comparison of smokers and non-smokers. Non-smokers live, on the average, 10 years longer than smokers, and thus their death rates would be shown in curve B, while death rates for smokers would be shown in curve A. The increased damage from the smokers' environment causes an overall increase in the death risk without altering the aging process, that is whatever process causes the exponential increase in death risk with increasing age.

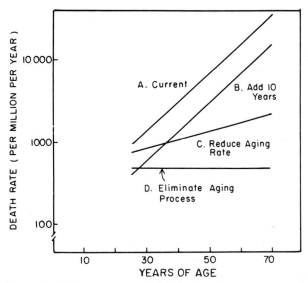

Fig. 1.2. Simplified curves are used to illustrate the effects on the total death rate, curve A (taken from deaths from all causes in Fig. 1.1), of the following: curve B – adding 10 years life expectancy; curve C – greatly reducing the rate of aging; and curve D – eliminating the aging process.

Line C in Fig. 1.2 illustrates the effect of reducing the aging rate, so that the death risk increases more slowly with increasing age. The results illustrated in line C show a major reduction in the aging rate. Line D illustrates the relationship between death risk and age if there was no aging process. The risk of death does not change throughout life.

Besides the increasing death risk, aging causes decreases in functional capacity for many different organ systems. These decreases usually appear to be linear rather than exponential. For many parameters, functional capacity changes very little in healthy individuals over most of their lifespans. For other types of functions, such as respiratory (maximum breathing capacity, vital capacity), and those depending on maximal blood-flow (which is impaired by cardio-vascular blockage as is renal plasma-flow) there may be declines of 50 per cent or more over the adult lifespan. Nevertheless, it is difficult to see how these relatively small linear declines in functional capacity can be responsible for a doubling in death risk every nine years.

CAUSES OF AGING

Gerontologists disagree as to whether a simple cause of aging exists. Many researchers believe that each tissue develops malfunctions as it wears out, at rates depending on each individual's unique combination of genotype and environment. However, an alternative possibility is that there are underlying causes of many of the malfunctions that develop with age. There are two types of evidence that help support this view; first, death risks from apparently unrelated diseases show parallel increases with age, as shown in Fig. 1.1. This suggests that underlying aging processes cause the increased vulnerability to all of these diseases. Second, certain types of living cells never seem to wear out, suggesting that aging is not inevitable. Some lines of tumour cells appear able to proliferate indefinitely, and the germ line, the normal cell types that form ova and sperm, must not age. Of course, neither tumour nor germ cells have to be like other body tissues. However, they illustrate that it is possible for mammalian cell types to avoid aging.

A wide variety of theories have been proposed to explain aging, and they tend to fall into two general classes: wear-and-tear, and programmed (Fig. 1.3). The two types of theories converge in the possibility that repair processes to minimize damage from wear-and-tear are programmed to decline with age. Wear-and-tear theories tend to be intrinsic, so that the aging of a tissue is caused by something internal. Programmed aging theories tend to be extrinsic so that the aging of a tissue is caused by something outside acting on it.

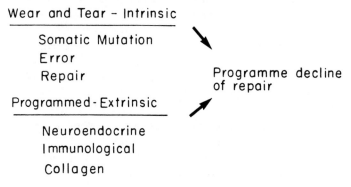

THEORIES OF AGING

Wear and Tear – Intrinsic
_____
    Somatic Mutation
    Error
    Repair   Programme decline
               of repair
Programmed - Extrinsic
_____
    Neuroendocrine
    Immunological
    Collagen

Fig. 1.3. Theories of aging fall into general classes, and this figure illustrates their relationships.

Wear-and-tear

Wear-and-tear theories are intuitively satisfying. Just as a machine cannot be designed and built to be used without eventually breaking down, neither can an organism. These theories may be applied at any level of biological organization. Functions of the whole individual, intact organs, tissues, cells, or the molecules in the cell may fail because of accumulating damage. With the recent revolutionary discoveries in molecular biology and genetics, modern wear-and-tear theories concentrate on the molecules making up the gene, the DNA.

The suggestion that aging is caused by accumulating somatic mutations is very popular. This theory was initially supported by Curtis (1963), who found that there were increasing percentages of cells with abnormal chromosomes in regenerating livers of older individuals, and that shorter-lived mouse strains showed a faster increase with age. At the same time, irradiation was found to shorten lifespans and increase damage to chromosomes, presumably as a result of somatic mutations. Together these observations suggested a very satisfying explanation for aging. During the lifespan, somatic cells gradually accumulate so much genetic damage that they cannot function correctly.

Further support for the somatic mutation theory of aging came from the realization that mutations can be caused by the highly reactive chemical intermediates, free radicals, that can be produced by inappropriate reactions with oxygen and other active molecules (Harman 1956). Furthermore, the increase in cancer incidence with age is explained if accumulations of mutations in certain cells cause them to become transformed into cancer cells. Evidence against the somatic mutation theory is the fact that germ cells apparently avoid aging, as previously mentioned, and sublethal doses of chemical mutagens have much less effect on longevity than would be expected from the numbers of mutations they cause. Furthermore, high-energy irradiation does not accelerate all aging processes at a constant rate.

Recently, strong support for the somatic mutation theory has come from studies showing that several types of repair mechanisms are more efficient in longer-lived species. Hart and Setlow (1974) found that DNA repair in fibroblasts exposed to ultraviolet light was much more extensive in cells from long-lived species. Richard Cutler and his colleagues (Tolmasoff *et al.* 1980) found that superoxide dismutase, an enzyme that removes oxygen radicals, has higher activity in livers, brains, and hearts of long-lived animals. When the enzyme levels are corrected for the rates of metabolism, amazingly good correlations with species longevity are obtained. These correlations are illustrated in Fig. 1.4 for a group of related primates that have a wide range of lifespans. Schwartz (1975) showed that higher amounts of enzymes to activate carcinogens are present in fibroblast cells from shorter-lived species. While his correlations are interesting, it is hard to interpret results in fibroblasts, since the enzymes that normally activate the type of carcinogen used are found in high concentrations in livers of all species. However, the combination of these different lines of evidence strongly suggests that mechanisms for repairing or preventing damage to DNA of somatic cells, are associated with lengthened species' lifespans.

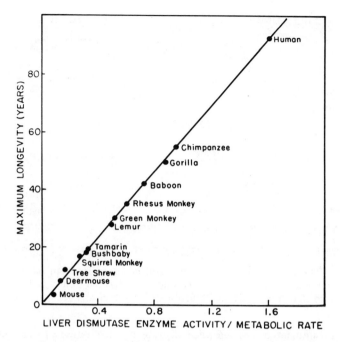

Fig. 1.4. The maximum longevities of two rodent and 11 primate species are plotted against superoxide dismutase enzyme activities in the liver (U/mg protein) divided by specific metabolic rates (calories/g per day) for each species. These data are given in Table 1 of Tolmasoff *et al.* (1980).

Programmed aging

Theories predicting that aging is programmed often suggest that aging results from the cell's functioning in a complex system. In these types of theories, changes with age are not necessarily internal within the cell types that malfunction. The functions of a single organ – perhaps a gland – may change with age and cause extensive changes in the internal environment of the aging individual. These changes may cause malfunctions in many other tissues, and the gland may be programmed to cause these malfunctions. Tissues that malfunction as a result of exposure to the environment of the aging animal, would function normally if transplanted into the normal environment of a young animal (Fig. 1.5). Systemic theories, therefore, lead to optimistic predictions about health benefits. Rather than having to restore the DNA of every malfunctioning cell, we would only need to clean up their environment.

It is possible that neuroendocrine changes initiate many parts of the aging process. Finch and his colleagues (1980) have reviewed studies suggesting that there are interactions between the ovaries and the hypothalamic–pituitary axis that cause reproductive aging in mice, and may cause it in all mammals. Although the number of oocytes in the ovary declines dramatically over the adult lifespan, this does not seem to be the primary cause for the loss of female reproductive ability with age, as shown by the following experiments. If young

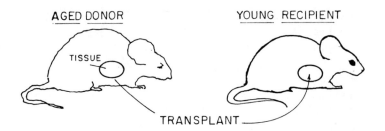

AGED DONOR   YOUNG RECIPIENT

TISSUE

TRANSPLANT

AGED ENVIRONMENT   *HEALTHY ENVIRONMENT*

POSSIBILITY   RESULT

A. AGING INTRINSIC IN ALL CELLS   DEFECT CONTINUES

B. AGING TIMED BY ONE CRUCIAL TISSUE DEFECT CURED

C. AGING RESULTS FROM INTERACTION   DEFECT CURED

Fig. 1.5.   The possible results of transplanting tissue from an old donor into a young recipient are illustrated. It is assumed that the donor and recipient are syngeneic so that tissue grafts will not be immunologically rejected.

ovaries are implanted into old mice, there is no resumption of oestrous cycles. However, if the old recipients had been ovariectomized when young, and then, after they had grown old, were the recipients of young ovaries, the old animals would show normal oestrous cycles. This suggests that the regular cycling of the ovaries over the lifespan causes a loss in the ability of the hypothalamic–pituitary axis to interact with the young ovary and cause cycling. Corresponding experiments have shown that ovaries from old individuals of certain strains that had long passed their reproductive lifespan still could function normally enough to produce healthy offspring after transplantation into young recipients.

Finch *et al.* (1980) postulated that there is a limited degree of oestrogen exposure that an individual can endure before oestrous cycles cease. This exposure may result from normal cycling over the lifespan, or may be induced by artificial injection of large amounts of oestrogens, which have been shown to cause irregular cycling and loss of cycling at a greatly accelerated rate.

It is possible that the loss of reproductive ability in females is controlled by mechanisms similar to those that control other aging processes that occur later in life. If this is true, the endocrine controls may be under feedback regulation, so that the effects of operating the target organ cause the controlling parts of the neuroendocrine system to decline in functional ability, as seems to be the case with the ovary, the target organ controlled by the hypothalamic–pituitary axis. The mechanism causing this decline is not known for this system, nor is it known whether the decline can be reversed.

The most controversial work in neuroendocrine control of the aging process has been done by Denckla (1978), and has exciting implications. Even if incorrect, these studies illustrate the possibilities opened up by studies of neuroendocrine aging. Denckla found evidence that a previously unknown hormone produced by the pituitary causes the rate of metabolism (burning food as fuel) to decrease with age. When Denckla removed pituitary glands from old rats and gave them supplements to replace necessary pituitary functions, the rats appeared younger and more energetic, and immune responses and many of their other functions returned to youthful levels. While many died young, presumably from endocrine imbalances, the longest-lived treated rats outlived the longest-lived controls. Denckla suggests that many aging processes are controlled by this pituitary hormone.

This suggestion is extremely exciting, but Denckla's work must be repeated by other investigators before it is widely accepted. If it is true, many of the problems that occur with age might be alleviated by finding a way to halt or retard production of a single factor in the pituitary. I have done preliminary studies of pituitary removal in aging mice, and found that some of Denckla's results were repeatable in the mouse, and others were not. This system is certainly interesting enough for further study, but extremely careful work will be necessary to fully evaluate the importance of pituitary factors in aging.

TRANSPLANTATION EXPERIMENTS

One way of testing whether a particular tissue ages intrinsically (Fig. 1.3) is to do the transplantation experiments illustrated in Fig. 1.5. If tissues that malfunction in old individuals show normal function after transplantation to young recipients, then the tissues have not aged intrinsically. A variety of different types of tissues have been tested in this manner. Geiringer (1954) understood the importance of distinguishing intrinsically timed changes in an organ from changes induced by the aging animal's internal environment. He showed that transplanted adrenocortical tissue could function for at least three years, while supporting normal growth and reproduction. This was a few months longer than his rats lived, but not longer than the maximum possible rat lifespan. Krohn (1966) also used this system and fully explained how it could be interpreted. He showed that old ovaries sometimes were capable of supporting successful pregnancies in young recipients, and that transplanted skin was capable of outliving its donor. His longest-lived mouse skin-graft was 6.7 years old, about twice as long as the maximum mouse lifespan. Unfortunately, no functional tests were reported, and there was no way to prove that the functioning cells in the skin had, in fact, come from the original donor and had not migrated to the skin from successive recipients.

The problem of identifying donor cells is less critical in grafts of complex organs, such as the kidney. Recently, a 75-year-old human kidney transplant successfully supported its recipient through the trauma of giving birth, according to a report by Carolyn B. Coulam of the Mayo Clinic to the 1981 Clinical Congress of the American College of Surgeons. This suggests that human kidneys behave in the same way as did the rat kidneys studied by Hollander and his colleagues (1971; van Bezooijen et al. 1974). These workers found a maximum rat kidney lifespan of 46 months, while the longest lived rat of the strain used lived for 39 months. Since a single transplanted kidney had to replace both kidneys of the recipient, the functional capacity of the old kidney was tested rigorously. Unfortunately, even 46 months is close enough to the maximum rat lifespan so that renal aging may be intrinsic, but just a little slower in some cases than the aging process that causes death in the intact individual.

Cellular aging

Systemic aging theories were strongly supported when it was believed that chick-embryo fibroblasts raised in tissue culture were immortal, because they could continue proliferating without limit. This view was popular for 40 years, until the 1960s. People assumed that somatic cells generally could be immortal, if they weren't part of a system whose function declined. Hayflick (1965, 1968) challenged these ideas, when he showed that normal fibroblasts in tissue culture have a limited proliferative capacity. Only transformed cells proliferated without limit, and those showed many characteristics of cancer cells rather than normal cells. Hayflick proposed that the loss of proliferative capacity in tissue cultures was cellular aging, and many people adopted it as a model system in which to study the aging process.

The system has been questioned for several reasons. There is only a small difference between old and young adults in the proliferative capacity of their fibroblasts. The loss of proliferative capacity may result from cell differentiation to non-proliferating forms rather than from aging. Moreover, there is no evidence that anyone ages because their fibroblasts or any other cells exhaust their proliferative capacity.

My first experiments in this area were designed to test whether cell types in animals behaved like Hayflock's fibroblasts. I compared haemopoietic stem-cell lines from old and young mice and tested their ability to carry out normal functions. Throughout the lifespan of the individual in which they grow, these stem-cell lines must proliferate and differentiate. They continuously form red blood cells and other short-lived blood and lymphoid cell types. I transplanted old stem-cells into young animals and studied their ability to perform these functions.

Figure 1.5 shows the possible results and interpretations from experiments in which old cells are transplanted into young recipients. If aging is intrinsic in the transplanted cells, their functional defect that developed with age will continue. However, if aging is timed by a different tissue, the functional defect will be cured in the healthy young recipient. This will also happen if aging results from interactions of many tissues with age.

In my experiments, stem-cell lines from healthy old donors functioned as well as those from young donors. They repopulated stem-cell-deficient recipients and produced differentiated cells (Harrison 1973). Mouse marrow-cell lines were able to continue functioning normally for several times as long as a mouse lives (Fig. 1.6), with some functioning for more than eight years (Harrison 1979). These experiments were limited by the numbers of serial transplantations possible. All cell lines lost some of their ability to develop normally (measured by curing anaemic W/W^v mice) as they were serially transplanted (Fig. 1.6). Most died out after five to six serial transplantations (Harrison 1975, 1979).

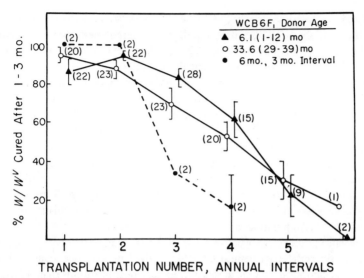

Fig. 1.6. Results of serial transplantation of mouse bone-marrow at 300- to 550-day intervals are given. Young genetically anaemic W/W^v recipients were repopulated and cured by the transplanted normal marrow, if it functioned normally. Donor ages are given in the top panel as mean (range) when the marrow was first transplanted. The number of cured, healthy donors used at each transplantation is in parentheses with a mean of 4.5 (range 2 to 11) young W/W^v recipients per donor. Each point is the mean value for those donors, and brackets enclose ± one standard error. (These data formed a portion of Figure 1 in Harrison (1979).)

Function, identification, and control

These experiments met the three criteria of function, identification, and control. Aging was determined by the ability to function normally. This was tested by curing genetically-anaemic mice, by saving the lives of lethally-irradiated recipients, and by supporting normal recovery after severe bleeding (Harrison 1973, 1975). Cells were identified by genetic markers of three kinds: the W/W^v anaemia of the recipients, differing haemoglobin from the recipients, and the T6 chromosome translocation marker. As controls, young and old tissues were transplanted in identical experiments, and they were compared directly (Harrison 1973, 1975, 1979). Furthermore, old donors usually did not have diseases that were transplanted with the stem cells. In cases where this did happen, tumour cell precursors were transplanted, and all the recipients of the marrow-cell line from the diseased donor died early with leukaemia-like cancers (Harrison 1975).

When performing transplantation experiments to determine whether tissues are intrinsically defective as a result of aging, it is important to meet the following criteria: (i) aging should be measured by loss of functional ability; (ii) the transplanted tissues should be unambiguously identified; (iii) old tissues should be compared with identically-treated young controls; (iv) the old donor should not have any diseases that will permanently affect the tissues. These criteria can be met in studies of stem cells, and in further experiments we have tested the lymphoid stem-cell lines that populate the immune system. These may be descended from the same stem-cell lines that populate the haemopoietic system. Initially we found that recipients populated with stem cells from old and young donors gave similar immune responses. Even when the immune responses of the original old donors were lowered, the recipients that had been repopulated by the stem-cell lines from old and young donors gave similar responses (Harrison *et al.* 1977).

In order to maximize potential differences between the functional ability of old and young stem-cell lines, we mixed stem cells from old or young donors with genetically-distinguishable cells from a pool of young donors. These mixtures were transplanted into genetically-distinguishable recipients. In these cases the mixed stem cells compete to repopulate the recipients, and small defects in repopulating ability are greatly magnified. We did not find significant differences between old and young stem-cell lines, but a single serial transplantation greatly reduced their repopulating ability (Harrison *et al.* 1978). The stem-cell lines from old and young mice were capable of functioning normally for a maximum of five or six serial transplantations (Fig. 1.6). Our evidence suggested that a single transplantation caused at least four and possibly more than 10 times as much damage as a lifetime of normal functioning. Thus, it appears that stem-cell lines are capable of functioning normally for at least 20 lifespans. If they did not have to be transplanted as the recipients grew old, they might be immortal.

FUTURE RESEARCH IN AGING

Comfort (1979) has often suggested that we should develop accurate measures of physiological age, and has listed criteria that should be met by such measures. While this is an essential development, initially such measures will be particularly valuable in laboratory mice and rats. Treatments to alter aging rates can most easily be developed in these species, because they age 30 times faster than human beings, and can be studied under well-defined conditions. However, a severe block to more rapid progress in understanding and alleviating the aging process, is the absence of a good test to determine whether a treatment affects the aging rate. As things now stand, the only such test we have is longevity.

Consider the traditional procedures followed to assay mammalian aging for the purpose of evaluating a treatment that may alter the aging process. To use the longevity test, we treat a minimum of 30 mice or rats, and also have an equal number of controls. The assay takes 2–3 years, as long as the animals live. Progress is bound to be slow when it takes this long to learn what happened in an experiment. Moreover, longevity is not a reliable measure. It is easily affected by many environmental factors. It is grossly defective as a sole endpoint, because it only tests the first system that malfunctions enough to kill the animal. It would give positive results if a treatment kept animals alive longer but in poorer health, although this is not what we want to do. Assaying solely for longevity fails to detect treatments that improve the health of non-vital systems without extending longevities. Yet such treatments might relieve great amounts of human suffering.

To develop a more useful assay for aging, physiological changes should be measured in as many different systems as possible. This would allow us to analyse general patterns of health, rather than basing results only on whatever kills the animal the soonest, as is the case when longevity is the assay. Furthermore, many reliable physiological changes occur in a shorter time than the entire lifespan. These should be detectable in less than 10 years in man, or four months in mice or rats, thus leading to a much faster and more precise assay than longevity. Of course, longevity and pathology (what appears to be wrong with the animal) at death must be measured whenever possible; these parameters are essential components of assays for physiological age. They also will show how the old and new assays of aging are related.

Psychopharmacologists should be able to provide valuable input in developing effective assays for physiological age. Some of the most important changes with aging are in mental functions, and the changes in these that are most relevant to man are difficult to measure in rodents. It would be useful to have a reliable test that could demonstrate memory losses in laboratory mice and rats over their lifespans. Of course such tests should not permanently affect the animals and should be as easy to do as possible. Although tests showing changes with age in short-term memory have been reported, there is conflicting information on how repeatable they are. If old animals have poorer memories than young ones, it should be possible to develop a test that demonstrates this over a range of conditions. The test should work even when performed by people who are not researchers in animal behaviour. It would be interesting to determine how aging of apparently unrelated systems, such as collagen, renal function, immune response, metabolic rate, strength, reflex time, and memory are cor-ordinated. However, to co-ordinate them, the same individuals must be measured. Usually this means that a wide variety of tests must be run in a single laboratory, so the tests should be as simple as possible.

I have tried to illustrate some theories of aging and some tests of these theories. I have not offered a theory because I don't think there is enough reliable evidence. At this point we cannot predict how long it will take researchers to learn enough to be able to beneficially affect the aging process. Nevertheless, I believe that research in aging should be vigourously pursued, because the potential payoff in terms of human health is so great. Most ill health in economically developed areas is a direct result of the aging process. Even if the basic aging process cannot be altered, it should be possible to develop treatments that reduce the discomforts of old age.

Acknowledgements

These studies were supported in part by National Institutes of Health Research Grants AG-01755 and AG-00594 from the National Institute on Aging, and AM-25687 from the National Institute of Arthritis, Diabetes, and Digestive and Kidney Diseases. I am indebted to Clinton M. Astle, Jon Archer, and Joan D. DeLaittre for dependable technical assistance. The drawings in this chapter were produced by Ruth Soper of the Jackson Laboratory Art and Photography Department.

REFERENCES

Comfort, A. (1979) *The biology of senescence*, 3rd edn. Elsevier, New York.

Curtis, H. J. (1963). Biological mechanisms underlying the aging process. *Science, NY* **141**, 686-94.

Denckla, W. D. (1978). Interactions between age and the neuroendocrine and immune systems. *Fed. Proc. Fedn Am. Socs exp. Biol.* **37**, 1263-7.

Finch, C. E., Felicio, L. S., Flurkey, K., Gee, D. M., Mobbs, C., Nelson, J. F., and Osterburg, H. H. (1980). Studies on ovarian-hypothalamic-pituitary interactions during reproductive aging in C57BL/6J mice. *Peptides* **1**, Suppl. 1, 163-75.

Geiringer, E. (1954). Homotransplantation as a method of gerontologic research. *J. Geront.* **9**, 142-9.

Harman, D. (1956). Aging – a theory based on free radical and radiation chemistry. *J. Geront.* **11**, 298-300.

Harrison, D. E. (1973). Normal production of erythrocytes by mouse marrow continuous for 73 months. *Proc. natn Acad. Sci. USA* **70**, 3184-8.

— (1975). Normal function of transplanted marrow cell lines from aged mice. *J. Geront.* **30**, 279-85.

— (1979). Mouse erythropoietic stem cell lines function normally 100 months: loss related to number of transplantations. *Mechan. Aging Devl.* **9**, 427-33.

—, Astle, C. M., and DeLaittre, J. A. (1978). Loss of proliferative capacity in immunohemopoietic stem cells caused by serial transplantation rather than aging. *J. exp. Med.* **147**, 1526-31.

— — and Doubeday, J. W. (1977). Stem cell lines from old immunodeficient donors give normal responses in young recipients. *J. Immun.* **118**, 1223-7.

Hart, R. W. and Setlow, R. B. (1974). Correlation between deoxyribonucleic acid excision-repair and life-span in a number of mammalian species. *Proc. natn Acad. Sci. USA* **71**, 2169-73.

Hayflick, L. (1965). The limited *in vitro* lifetime of human diploid cell strains. *Expl Cell Res.* **37**, 614-36.

— (1968). Human cells and aging. *Scient. Am.* **218**, 32-7.

Hollander, C. F. (1971). Age limit for the use of any geneic donor kidneys in the rat. *Transplant. Proc.* **3**, 594-7. (Also see the article by Van Bezooijen *et al.*, below.)

Kohn, R. R. (1978). *Principles of mammalian aging*, 2nd edn. Prentice-Hall, Englewood Cliffs, NJ.

Krohn, P. L. (1962). Heterochronic transplantation in the study of aging. *Proc. R. Soc.* **B157**, 128-47.

— (1966). Transplantation and aging. In *Topics in the biology of aging* (ed. P. L. Krohn) pp. 125-48. Wiley, New York.

Schwartz, A. E. (1975). Correlation between species lifespan and ability to activate 7,12 dimethylbenz-d-anthracene to a form mutagenic to a mammalian cell. *Expl Cell Res.* **44**, 445-7.

Tolmasoff, J., Ono, T., and Cutler, R. G. (1980). Superoxide dismutase: correlation with life-span and specific metabolic rate in primate species. *Proc. natn Acad. Sci. USA* **77**, 2777-81.

van Beezooijen, K. F. A., deLeeuw-Israel, F. R., and Hollander, C. F. (1974). Long-term functional aspects of syngeneic orthotopic rat kidney grafts of different ages. *J. Geront.* **29**, 11-19.

2

Dementia and unconventional slow infections

MOIRA E. BRUCE AND A. G. DICKINSON

A major limitation in investigations into Alzheimer's dementia has been the lack of satisfactory animal models. In recent years a number of parallels have been recognized between Alzheimer's disease and scrapie, an infectious neurological disease of sheep (Dickinson et al. 1979). Both are slow diseases which follow a progressive and unremitting course. In each case pathological lesions are confined to the central nervous system and are degenerative in nature, with little or no evidence of inflammation or demyelination. Most significantly, some of the characteristic pathological features of Alzheimer's disease can be reproduced by infecting particular strains of mouse with particular strains of scrapie (Table 2.1). These scrapie models now make it possible to study neuropathological changes of the type seen in Alzheimer's disease under controlled experimental conditions, as well as providing opportunities for testing pharmacological treatments which might modify the development of these lesions.

SCRAPIE

Scrapie is caused by an unconventional infectious agent (a 'virino': Dickinson and Outram 1979) which, although its molecular nature remains unproved, can be regarded as a small virus-like organism. The disease can be transmitted to mice from most natural sheep cases, using inocula prepared from brain or lympho-reticular tissue. By serially passaging scrapie isolates in mice many distinct strains of agent have been separated, identified primarily on the basis of their incubation periods in known mouse genotypes (Dickinson and Fraser 1977). A range of lesions is seen in the brain, the occurrence and severity of which differ according to the agent strain, mouse strain and route of infection, each combination producing a characteristic pattern of pathological change (Fraser 1979). Although none of these combinations reproduces the full range of changes seen in Alzheimer's disease, certain lesions characteristic of Alzheimer's disease have been identified in particular murine scrapie models; firstly, the presence of amyloid-containing plaques in the brain, secondly, a deficit in the cholinergic neurotransmitter system and, thirdly, the selective loss of neurons, particularly the pyramidal neurons of the hippocampus.

Amyloid plaques

In the case of Alzheimer's disease, amyloid foci occur in the brain in the form of senile plaques which are seen in large numbers in patients with this type of dementia and in smaller numbers in non-demented elderly people. Cerebral

TABLE 2.1.   *Characteristics of Alzheimer's disease and scrapie. Unbroken lines indicate consistent features; broken lines indicate that the occurrence varies between cases or models.*

	Alzheimer's disease	Murine scrapie — With high incidence of cerebral amyloid	Murine scrapie — Other forms
Incubation period (extraneural infection route)	Not applicable or unknown		
Age at onset	Middle to late life	*Half lifespan to 'beyond' normal lifespan; *Early-middle to late life	*Quarter lifespan to 'beyond' normal lifespan
Interval between first signs and terminal phase	4–10 years	*2–10 months	
Duration of terminal phase	6 months	3–8 weeks	2–8 weeks
Clinico-pathological features	Progressive encephalopathy		
Neurochemical changes	Depression of choline acetyl transferase		
Neuropathological changes	Granulovacuolar degeneration; Neurofibrillary tangles; Argyrophilic senile or amyloid plaques; Other forms of cerebral amyloid; Vacuolar degeneration of grey matter; Neuronal loss and glial reaction; Some suggestions of asymmetry; Vacuolar degeneration in white matter; No demyelination or inflammatory pathology	Frequent asymmetry	No asymmetry

*Details depend on host genotype, agent strain, route, and dose.

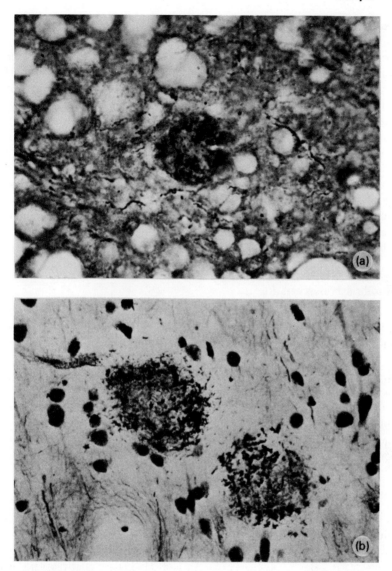

Fig. 2.1.   Amyloid-containing plaques demonstrated by silver staining (a) in murine scrapie (Bodian × 600) and (b) in Alzheimer's disease (von Braunmühl × 400). (Alzheimer slide was provided by Professor B. E. Tomlinson.)

amyloid plaques have also been seen in mice injected with most scrapie isolates (Fig. 2.1). Their frequency, like the severity of other scrapie lesions, depends on the strain of agent, strain of mouse, and route of inoculation, some agent strains producing large numbers of plaques in all mouse genotypes, some producing moderate numbers and others producing none (Bruce *et al.* 1976). The plaques in scrapie and Alzheimer's disease are closely similar in structure, consisting of an amyloid core surrounded by microglia and degenerating neuronal processes

(Bruce and Fraser 1975; Wisniewski *et al.* 1975). At present, infection with scrapie is the only experimental model for amyloid-containing senile plaques.

In mice amyloid plaques have only been seen in association with scrapie infection; they have not been identified in uninfected old mice (Dayan 1971; Bruce and Fraser 1982). On the other hand, senile plaques, which are seen in about 80 per cent of non-demented octogenarians, are regarded as a 'normal' aging change in man (Tomlinson 1979) and similar structures have also been found in old animals of several other mammalian species (Wisniewski and Terry 1973). Therefore amyloid-containing plaques may not necessarily be restricted to 'disease' processes as these are usually defined. However, there has been great difficulty in the past in finding a satisfactory experimental model for senile plaques, suggesting that this type of structure can result from only a limited number of stimuli. Amyloid plaques in scrapie and Alzheimer's disease may not share the same primary cause, but it is probable that the sequence of events leading to their formation in each case is basically similar.

Neurofibrillary degeneration

The other major histopathological lesion of Alzheimer's disease, neurofibrillary degeneration, has not been seen in any of our scrapie models, although it has been reported to occur in some cases of Creutzfeldt–Jakob disease, a recognized analogue of scrapie in man (McMenemy 1963). Neurofibrillary tangles occur in several other human neurological diseases (Iqbal *et al.* 1977) and are present in the brains of the majority of non-demented old people, but they have never been identified in any species other than man. Their absence in murine scrapie might simply reflect this restriction to the human species. Granulovacuolar degeneration, which is frequent in Alzheimer's disease and appears to be a 'normal' aging change in man, has also not been identified in murine scrapie.

Cholinergic deficit

It is well established that, in Alzheimer's disease, there is a significant reduction in the activity of choline acetyl transferase (CAT) and acetylcholinesterase, enzymes involved in the cholinergic neurotransmitter system (Davies and Moloney 1976; Bowen *et al.* 1976). This deficit is particularly severe in the cerebral cortex, amygdala, and hippocampus, areas of brain in which senile plaques and neurofibrillary tangles are also particularly frequent. As comparable changes do not occur in enzymes associated with other neurotransmitter systems, the depression of cholinergic activity has been interpreted as being due to the selective loss of cholinergic neurons or their nerve endings. A similar reduction in CAT activity has been reported in C57BL mice infected with various strains of scrapie, including those which do not produce amyloid plaques (McDermott *et al.* 1978). This lack of correlation between the occurrence of plaques and the CAT deficit in scrapie is surprising, in view of the fact that a negative correlation has been demonstrated between CAT levels and senile plaque counts in the neocortex in demented and non-demented humans (Perry 1979).

Neuronal loss

Widespread neuronal loss is not a characteristic feature of murine scrapie, although it is possible that there is a marginal dropout which remains unrecognized. However, some cases show an obvious loss of pyramidal neurons in the hippocampus, accompanied by a glial reaction (Fig. 2.2) (Fraser 1979a,b). This change may be similar to the degenerative pathology seen in the hippocampus in a high proportion of Alzheimer patients (Corsellis 1970). In murine scrapie the

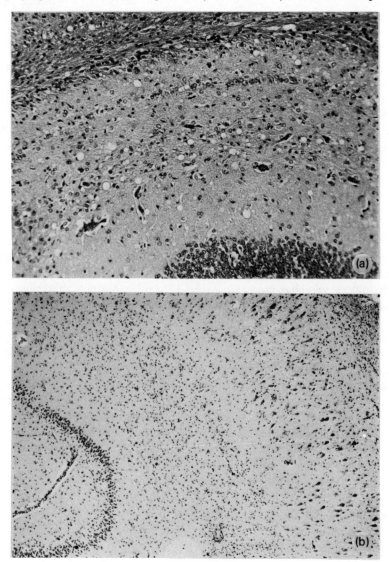

Fig. 2.2. Loss of hippocampal pyramidal neurons (a) in murine scrapie (H & E × 100) and (b) in Alzheimer's disease (Nissl × 40). (Alzheimer slide was provided by Professor B. E. Tomlinson.)

lesion is seen with a wide range of agent and mouse strains, but is particularly severe in certain combinations injected intracerebrally, not necessarily in association with amyloid plaques or a CAT deficit.

In certain other scrapie models an intense gliosis is seen in the thalamus, similar to that associated with neuronal loss in the hippocampus. It is likely that this gliosis is also secondary to selective neuronal loss, although this change is difficult to quantify because of the more complicated architecture of the thalamus.

ALZHEIMER'S DISEASE

Using the appropriate scrapie models it is now possible to produce experimentally most of the characteristic lesions of Alzheimer's disease. It must be stressed that the most suitable scrapie model for each of these lesions is different, suggesting that they are not necessarily interdependent. The great advantage of these models is that the development of the lesions can be traced, with reference to a known starting point, the date of injection, and a known clinical scrapie end-point. The identification of experimental variables which modify this development will greatly contribute towards understanding the mechanisms involved. In addition it may be possible to identify pharmacological treatments which either prevent or reverse the lesions, and which could eventually lead to the development of therapeutic treatments for Alzheimer's disease. A crucial question is therefore whether any of these changes is in fact reversible.

Senile plaques

In Alzheimer's disease a correlation has been found between the degree of dementia and the number of senile plaques in the brain (Blessed *et al.* 1968). Many of the neuronal processes involved in senile plaques, although grossly abnormal, still retain intact synaptic connections (Terry and Wisniewski 1970) and it is possible that functional deficits resulting from the presence of senile plaques are potentially reversible. In scrapie amyloid plaques are often seen in the white matter, suggesting that nerve terminals are not necessarily involved in plaque formation and therefore that amyloid deposition is the primary event (Bruce and Fraser 1981). The chemical nature and origin of the amyloid protein are not yet known, but it may be possible to find treatments which will prevent its accumulation in the brain. Most of the amyloid plaques appear during the last quarter of the scrapie incubation period, at a time when other histological lesions can also be detected (Bruce 1981). It is known that experimental variables operating at the time of initial infection with scrapie, such as route of inoculation and dilution of inoculum, profoundly influence the numbers and distribution of plaques eventually produced (Bruce and Fraser 1981). Treatments which will modify plaque production once infection has been established have yet to be identified.

Hippocampal lesions

The loss of hippocampal pyramidal neurons, accompanied by a proliferation of glial elements, occurs relatively late in the scrapie incubation period (Fraser and Scott, unpublished observation). Within a single experimental group there is often great variation between individuals in the occurrence and extent of this loss, suggesting that it may not be an inevitable consequence of scrapie infection in these models. Understanding the basis of this variation is important for two reasons. Firstly, a similar pathology in the hippocampus occurs in temporal lobe epilepsy, hypoglycaemia, and anoxia, and can be induced with a variety of neuroactive amino acids and peptides (McGeer and McGeer 1981; Diemer and Siemkowicz 1981; Nadler *et al*. 1978; Corsellis 1970). Secondly, it has been shown that, in scrapie, vacuolar degeneration in the presence of an otherwise intact pyramidal layer precedes the neuronal loss in the hippocampus; it has therefore been suggested that this represents the development of the pathological process from a reversible step to an irreversible one (Fraser 1979*a,b*). One interesting aspect of this hippocampal lesion is the intense astrocytic mitosis seen at an early stage of its development (Fraser and Scott, unpublished observation), leading to Alzheimer type II astrocytic metaplasia which accompanies the terminal stage (Fraser 1976*b*). This suggests a local disorder in ammonia detoxification by the astrocyte-specific glutamine synthetase enzyme (Martinez-Hernandez *et al*. 1977).

Prevention of cholinergic deficit

Preliminary work suggests that the cholinergic deficit seen with several scrapie models also occurs only in the terminal stages of the disease (McDermott, personal communication). Choline therapy has not convincingly been found to be effective in alleviating the symptoms of Alzheimer's disease (Glen and Whalley 1979). Pharmacological treatments aimed at preventing, rather than supplementing, the deficit can now be tested using the appropriate scrapie models.

AETIOLOGY

The growing number of parallels which have been found between Alzheimer's disease and murine scrapie have important implications as they raise the possibility, however remote, that an infectious agent similar to scrapie might be aetiologically involved in Alzheimer's disease. Scrapie belongs to a small group of infective neurological diseases, caused by similar agents, which also includes Creutzfeldt–Jakob disease in man. Although Alzheimer's disease and Creutzfeldt–Jakob disease are usually distinguished on clinical and neuropathological criteria, some cases show characteristics of both diseases. In Alzheimer's disease there is little or no spongy vacuolation of the type usually seen in scrapie and related diseases. However, as there are some scrapie models in which vacuolar degeneration is minimal or absent, this should not necessarily exclude Alzheimer's disease from the group. In considering the possibility that a wider range of neurological diseases than now recognized might be caused by scrapie-like agents, it is important to stress the pathological diversity of scrapie in mice. Simply by changing the strain of agent or genotype of mouse, we can predictably produce specific types of pathology from an extremely wide range. It is possible that such strain variation also exists in related agents affecting man and, in the genetically heterogeneous human population, a wide range of pathology would be expected.

On the other hand, even if it is proved that some cases now diagnosed as Alzheimer's disease are caused by agents similar to scrapie, there is no reason to assume that Alzheimer's disease invariably has an infectious aetiology. The parallels with scrapie and with 'normal' aging might simply reflect the limited number of ways in which the nervous system can degenerate over extended periods of time. Whether or not Alzheimer's disease has an infectious aetiology, the murine models described here provide a promising experimental approach towards the understanding of the degenerative pathology of Alzheimer's disease and other little understood conditions of the central nervous system.

REFERENCES

Blessed, G., Tomlinson, B. E., and Roth, M. (1968). The association between quantitative measures of dementia and of senile change in the cerebral grey matter of elderly subjects. *Br. J. Psychiat.* **114**, 797–811.

Bowen, D. M., Smith, C. B., White, P., and Davison, A. N. (1976). Neurotransmitter-related enzymes and indices of hypoxia in senile dementia and other abiotrophies. *Brain* **99**, 459–96.

Bruce, M. E. (1981). Serial studies on the development of cerebral amyloidosis and vacuolar degeneration in murine scrapie. *J. comp. Path.* **91**, 589–97.

— Dickinson, A. G., and Fraser, H. (1976). Cerebral amyloidosis in scrapie in the mouse: effect of agent strain and mouse genotype. *Neuropath. appl. Neurobiol.* **2**, 471–8.

— and Fraser, H. (1975). Amyloid plaques in the brains of mice infected with scrapie: morphological variation and staining properties. *Neuropath. appl. Neurobiol.* **1**, 189–202.

— — (1981). Effect of route of infection on the frequency and distribution of cerebral amyloid plaques in scrapie mice. *Neuropath. appl. Neurobiol.* **7**, 289–98.

— — (1982). Effects of age on cerebral amyloid plaques in murine scrapie. *Neuropath. appl. Neurobiol.* **8**, 71–4.

Corsellis, J. A. N. (1970). The limbic areas in Alzheimer's disease and in other conditions associated with dementia. In *Alzheimer's disease and related conditions* (ed. G. E. W. Wolstenholme and M. O'Connor) pp. 37–45. Churchill, London.

Davies, P. and Moloney, A. J. F. (1976). Selective loss of central cholinergic neurons in Alzheimer's disease. *Lancet* ii, 1403.

Dayan, A. D. (1971). Comparative neuropathology of ageing: studies on the brains of 47 species of vertebrates. *Brain* **94**, 31–42.

Dickinson, A. G. and Fraser, H. (1977). Scrapie pathogenesis in inbred mice: an assessment of host control and response involving many strains of agent. In *Slow virus infections of the central nervous system* (ed. V. ter Meulen and M. Katz) pp. 3–14. Springer, New York.

— — and Bruce, M. E. (1979). Animal models for the dementias. In *Alzheimer's disease, early recognition of potentially reversible deficits* (ed. A. I. M. Glen and L. J. Whalley) pp. 42–5. Churchill Livingstone, Edinburgh.

— and Outram, G. W. (1979). The scrapie replication-site hypothesis and its implications for pathogenesis. In *Slow transmissible diseases of the nervous system* (ed. W. J. Hadlow and S. B. Prusiner) pp. 13–31. Academic Press, New York.

Diemer, N. H. and Siemkowicz, E. (1981). Regional neurone damage after cerebral ischaemia in the normo- and hypo-glycaemic rat. *Neuropath. appl. Neurobiol.* **7**, 217–27.

Fraser, H. (1979a). Neuropathology of scrapie: the precision of the lesions and their diversity. In *Slow transmissible diseases of the nervous system* (ed. W. J. Hadlow and S. B. Prusiner) pp. 387–406. Academic Press, New York.

— (1979b). The pathogenesis and pathology of scrapie. In *Aspects of slow and persistent virus infections* (ed. D. A. J. Tyrrell) pp. 30–58. Martinus Nijhoff, Hague.

Glen, A. I. M. and Whalley, L. J. (eds.) (1979). *Alzheimer's disease, early recognition of potentially reversible deficits.* Churchill Livingstone, Edinburgh.

Iqbal, K., Wisniewski, H. M., Grundke-Iqbal, I., and Terry, R. D. (1977). Neurofibrillary pathology: an update. In *The ageing brain and senile dementia* (ed. K. Nandy and I. Sherwin) pp. 209–27. Plenum Press, New York.

McDermott, J. R., Fraser, H., and Dickinson, A. G. (1978). Reduced cholineacetyltransferase activity in scrapie mouse brain. *Lancet* ii, 318–19.

McGeer, E. G. and McGeer, P. L. (1981). Neurotoxins as a tool in neurobiology. *Int. Rev. Neurobiol.* 22, 173–204.

McMenemy, W. H. (1963). The dementias and progressive diseases of the basal ganglia. In *Greenfield's neuropathology*, 2nd edn. pp. 520–76. Arnold, London.

Martinez-Hernandez, A., Bell, K. P., and Norenberg, M. D. (1977). Glutamine synthetase, glial localization in brain. *Science, NY* 195, 1356–8.

Nadler, J. V., Perry, B. W., and Cotman, C. W. (1978). Preferential vulnerability of hippocampus to intraventricular kainic acid. In *Kainic acid as a tool in neurobiology* (ed. E. G. McGeer, J. W. Olney, and P. L. McGeer) pp. 219–37. Raven Press, New York.

Perry, E. K. (1979). Correlations between psychiatric, neuropathological and biochemical findings in Alzheimer's disease. In *Alzheimer's disease, early recognition of potentially reversible deficits* (ed. A. I. M. Glen and L. J. Whalley) pp. 27–32. Churchill Livingstone, Edinburgh.

Terry, R. D. and Wisniewski, H. M. (1970). The ultrastructure of the neurofibrillary tangle and the senile plaque. In *Alzheimer's disease and related conditions* (ed. G. E. W. Wolstenholme and M. O'Connor) pp. 145–65. Churchill, London.

Tomlinson, B. E. (1979). The ageing brain. In *Recent advances in neuropathology*, No. 1, pp. 129–59. Churchill Livingstone, Edinburgh.

Wisniewski, H. M., Bruce, M. E., and Fraser, H. (1975). Infectious etiology of neuritic (senile) plaques in mice. *Science, NY* 190, 1108–10.

— and Terry, R. D. (1973). Reexamination of the pathogenesis of the senile plaque. In *Progress in neuropathology*, Vol. II (ed. H. M. Zimmerman) pp. 1–26. Grune and Stratton, New York.

3

Central neurotransmitters, memory, and dementia

T. J. CROW, A. J. CROSS, I. G. GROVE-WHITE, AND D. G. ROSS

The concept that specific central neurotransmitters play a role in memory processes has developed over the past 10 years. Most attention has focused upon acetylcholine, but some findings suggest that noradrenalin is also involved. Recently it has appeared that the functions of these neurochemical systems may be relevant to the pathology of memory – specifically in Alzheimer's type dementia and in Korsakoff's psychosis.

CHOLINERGIC MECHANISMS

Interest in the effects of drugs on learning processes dates from Gauss' (1906) description of 'twilight sleep' following the use of morphine and hyoscine in labour. More recent studies have focused on the amnesic properties of hyoscine when used as a premedicant. Hardy and Wakely (1962) found a 13 per cent incidence of amnesia for a simple visual stimulus following standard doses of hyoscine, compared to a 1 per cent incidence with atropine. Hyoscine and hyoscine–diazepam combinations have been found to impair recall of events immediately preceding anaesthesia (Pandit and Dundee 1970; Pandit *et al.* 1971).

These learning deficits have been validated in experimental studies. Safer and Allen (1971) found registration of new information (assessed as immediate recall) to be only mildly impaired following hyoscine 10 µg/kg, while after a 20-second delay there was gross impairment of recall. A comparison of hyoscine (scopolamine) with methscopolamine, which does not enter the central nervous system (CNS), established deficits of memory storage and cognitive non-memory tasks, following 1 mg of hyoscine, but no deficit of immediate memory (Drachman and Leavitt 1974). The pattern of cognitive and memory defects following hyoscine resembled that seen in a group of aged subjects. Other experiments (Ghoneim and Mewalt 1975; Petersen 1977) have established that the effects of hyoscine are primarily upon the acquisition of new information rather than its retrieval from a memory store.

Memory storage

There is substantial evidence that in normal memory storage two processes are involved, and that in some cases of the amnesic syndrome it is the transition from short-term (sometimes called primary) memory, to long-term (or secondary) memory that is impaired (Baddeley and Warrington 1970). A convenient technique for distinguishing these components is the free-recall test of Glanzer and Cunitz (1966). This technique has been used in a series of experiments designed to establish the point in the storage process at which hyoscine exerts its amnesic action (Crow and Grove-White 1973; Crow *et al*. 1976).

Subjects were presented with lists of 10 words, at a rate of one word per three seconds, and were asked to recall these words in any order, either immediately after presentation (immediate recall) or after 60 seconds of an interpolated task (delayed recall). When tested in this way subjects recall the later words in the immediate recall condition (the 'recency effect') much more frequently than the earlier words. In the delayed recall condition there is no preferential recall of later words. It is therefore suggested that the recency effect reflects the operation of short-term memory while long-term memory storage is seen in the findings on the 'non-recency' part of the immediate recall, and in the delayed recall condition. In the 60-second delay before recall in the latter condition, subjects were presented with random-letter sequences at a rate of one letter per second, and were asked to record alphabetical sequences (e.g. ab, st, mn, etc.). This task (the scanning task) has two functions – to prevent rehearsal and to provide a measure of information processing ability with a minimal learning component.

In the first experiment 12 subjects (aged 19 to 23 years) were submitted to the battery of tests on three occasions, receiving on each occasion hyoscine 0.4 mg, atropine 0.6 mg, or sodium chloride injection 1 ml, in a balanced design. As well as the free-recall and scanning tasks they were also required to complete a simple number–colour association learning task.

TABLE 3.1

	Immediate recall	Delayed recall	Number–colour associations	Scanning task
Maximum score	50	50	7	25
		mean correct responses ± 1 SEM		
Saline (1 ml)	27.9 ± 1.6	14.3 ± 1.3	7 ± 0	22.3 ± 1.2
Hyoscine (0.4 mg)	24.0 ± 1.3*	10.2 ± 1.3**	5.9 ± 0.5*	20.5 ± 1.1
Atropine (0.6 mg)	25.9 ± 1.3	14.1 ± 1.7	6.9 ± 0.1	20.3 ± 1.2

*$0.05 > p > 0.01$; **$0.001 > p$ vs saline.
From Crow and Grove-White (1973).

The results (Table 3.1) demonstrated significant deficits on each of the learning tasks (immediate and delayed recall and number–colour association) following hyoscine but not atropine, but no significant deficits following either drug on the information processing (scanning) task. An analysis of the results with respect to order of presentation of words within the 10-word lists (Fig. 3.1) revealed that there is little effect of hyoscine on that part of the curve attributed to short-term memory (the 'recency effect'), but that the amnestic influence of the drug was seen on the non-recency part of the immediate recall curve, and uniformly on the delayed recall curve.

The results therefore confirmed the selectivity of the action of hyoscine for learning processes and, together with previous findings (e.g. Safer and Allen

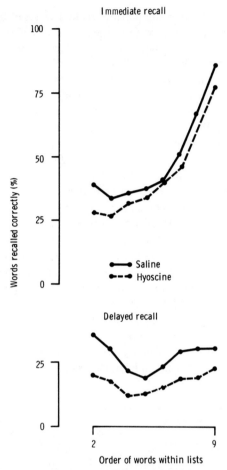

Fig. 3.1.   An analysis of the free-recall test results by order of presentation of words within the 10-word list (running totals, averaged over three positions at a time). (From Crow and Grove-White (1973).)

1971; Ghoneim and Mewalt 1975; Petersen 1977) suggested that this action was upon the transition from short-term to long-term memory, and not upon short-term acquisition or retrieval processes. The relative ineffectiveness of atropine in these experiments is consistent with the lower incidence of amnesia following atropine as premedication (Hardy and Wakely 1962) and may merely reflect the fact that central effects of atropine are generally seen only at higher doses (Longo 1966).

Hyoscine and other drugs

To determine whether the effects of hyoscine are specific to this drug, hyoscine was compared with amylobarbitone, diazepam, and chlorpromazine in the free-recall test (Crow *et al.* 1976).

The effects of chlorpromazine were substantial and were not confined to the

TABLE 3.2

	Maximum score	Saline	Chlorpromazine (12.5 or 25 mg)	Amylobarbitone (125 mg)	Diazepam (5 mg)	Hyoscine (0.4 mg)
Verbal learning						
Immediate recall	50	32.0 ± 1.2	$**25.3 \pm 1.8$	28.6 ± 2.2	27.9 ± 2.0	27.9 ± 2.5
Delayed recall	50	16.1 ± 2.0	$** 8.6 \pm 1.3$	15.3 ± 2.9	14.0 ± 2.6	$*10.6 \pm 1.4$
Scanning task	25	22.4 ± 1.6	$**16.4 \pm 1.4$	$*17.9 \pm 1.3$	20.4 ± 1.9	22.0 ± 1.5

$*p < 0.02$; $**p < 0.01$ for comparison with scores after saline.
From Crow *et al.* (1976).

learning task. Pulse-rate observations suggested that the intravenous administration of the drug was associated with significant cardiovascular effects and
these may have contributed to the surprisingly large impairments of test
performance. By contrast the effects of diazepam (5 mg) were insignificant.
There was, however, an interesting contrast between amylobarbitone (125 mg)
and hyoscine (0.4 mg), in that the former drug significantly impaired performance on the scanning task without significantly impairing free recall, while
hyoscine did not affect scanning-task performance but significantly impaired
delayed recall in the learning task. This contrast is particularly apparent when
the effects of these two drugs are examined in the order of presentation curves
in immediate and delayed recall (Fig. 3.2).

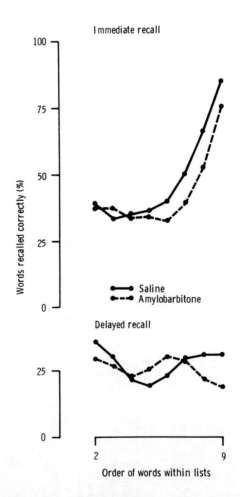

Fig. 3.2. Analysis of the free-recall test results by order of presentation of words,
within the 10-word list for (a) hyoscine 0.4 mg; and (b) amylobarbitone
(125 mg). (From Crow *et al.* (1976).)

TABLE 3.3. *The cholinergic system in Alzheimer's disease*

	Marker	Activity in AD (% control)	Reference
Presynaptic neuron	Cholineacetyltransferase (CAT)	51	Bowen *et al.* (1976)
		35	Davies and Maloney (1976)
		31	Perry *et al.* (1977)
		50	White *et al.* (1977)
		46	Bowen *et al.* (1979)
		(biopsy specimens)	
	Acetylcholinesterase (AChE)	17	Davies and Maloney (1976)
		50	Perry *et al.* (1981)
Postsynaptic neuron	Muscarinic receptor	100	Perry *et al.* (1977)
		100	Bowen *et al.* (1979)
		100	Davies and Verth (1978)
	Nicotinic receptor	80	Davies and Feisullin (1981)

Deficits in dementia

There is now a considerable amount of evidence to suggest that cholinergic mechanisms are deficient in senile dementia of the Alzheimer type (AD). Several groups of workers have reported that choline acetyltransferase, the enzyme responsible for the final step in the biosynthesis of acetylcholine, and a marker enzyme for cholinergic neurons, is reduced in AD. Acetyl cholinesterase, another marker of the presynaptic cholinergic neuron, is similarly reduced (Table 3.3). The observed reductions in these markers in AD appears to be greatest in some cortical areas and the hippocampus. In contrast, postsynaptic elements do not appear to be involved (Table 3.3). The reductions in choline acetyltransferase activity observed in AD correlate extremely well with the severity of dementia, as assessed by the mental test score (Perry *et al.* 1978). It seems possible that in the early stages of the disease process there is a relatively selective loss of cholinergic neurons. Since one of the most characteristic changes in AD is a loss of memory function, it appears that this may be directly related to a failure of cholinergic transmission.

The causation of AD remains obscure. It is of considerable interest, however, that the slow virus disease of sheep, known as scrapie (see previous chapter), which can be transmitted to the mouse has been found to be associated with neuropathological changes similar to those seen in AD (Wisniewski *et al.* 1975) and that in some species loss of choline acetyltransferase also occurs (McDermott *et al.* 1978; Table 3.4).

TABLE 3.4

Mice	Choline acetyltransferase		
	Forebrain	Mid-brain	Hindbrain
Control	21.4 ± 2.2	20.1 ± 1.0	19.8 ± 1.2
Semliki forest virus-infected	21.1 ± 1.8	26.5 ± 1.5	21.2 ± 1.4
Scrapie-infected	*15.5 ± 2.1	**13.2 ± 1.2	**12.1 ± 2.0

*$p < 0.05$; **$p < 0.01$.   From McDermott *et al.* (1978).

THE ROLE OF NORADRENALIN

Learning processes

A role for noradrenergic neurons in learning processes is also a possibility. The cerebral cortex and hippocampus are innervated by a diffuse network of noradrenalin-containing nerve terminals, and these originate from cell-bodies in the nucleus locus coeruleus in the mid-pontine region (Fig. 3.3).

Locus Coeruleus

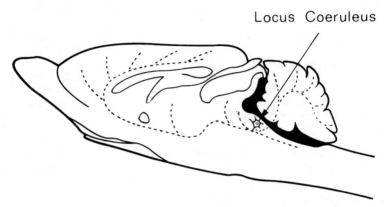

Fig. 3.3. The noradrenergic system arising from the locus coeruleus as described in the rat brain by Ungerstedt (1971).

There is evidence (Crow *et al.* 1972) that this system functions as part of a reward mechanism and it had previously been suggested (Crow 1968; Kety 1970) that the noradrenergic innervation of the cerebral cortex could be instrumental in converting short-term changes in intracortical synapses into the longer-term changes assumed to underly permanent memory. Pharmacological experiments have yielded findings consistent with a role for noradrenergic processes in memory storage. Thus diethyldithiocarbamate, an inhibitor of the noradrenalin-synthetic enzyme dopamine-β-hydroxylase, inhibits the acquisition of a passive avoidance response in rats (Randt *et al.* 1971). Moreover inhibition of passive avoidance learning is reported to be reversed by intraventricular administration of noradrenalin, provided such administration directly follows learning (Stein *et al.* 1975). This finding suggests a very specific role for noradrenalin and is consistent with the hypothesis described above which attributes to noradrenergic neurons the conversion of short- to long-term synaptic changes. Lesions of the locus coeruleus system itself have sometimes been reported as causing impairments of learning (Anlezark *et al.* 1973; Crow 1977). However, the interpretation of these experiments has been challenged on the grounds that similar impairments are not seen after neurochemical (i.e. 6-OH-dopamine-induced) rather than electrolytic lesions. Thus while intraventricularly administered 6-OH-dopamine has been reported to cause impaired learning of a complex motor task (Mason and Iversen 1975), a one-trial passive avoidance task (Rainbow *et al.* 1976) and a classically conditioned heart-rate response (Howard and Breese 1974), such deficits were not found when 6-OH-dopamine was injected into the noradrenalin-containing fibres ascending from the locus coeruleus to innervate the forebrain (Mason and Iversen 1975; Roberts *et al*. 1976). Moreover even though acquisition impairments were confirmed in some tasks (e.g. appetitive runway learning) after electrolytic lesions, these impairments did not seem to reflect a general learning deficit (Sessions *et al*. 1976). These findings have appeared damaging to the hypothesis that the locus coeruleus system is a necessary component in the mechanisms of learning.

Involvement of the locus coeruleus

However, these negative findings are not decisive. Thus to achieve complete electrolytic lesions of the locus coeruleus is surprisingly difficult and, while impaired learning occurs only with very extensive lesions (Crow 1977), it is by no means apparent that in those studies in which learning is reported as unimpaired (Amaral and Foss 1975; Sessions *et al*. 1976; Koob *et al*. 1978), complete bilateral ablations have been present. Moreover in the 6-OH-dopamine experiments only the ascending fibres have been lesioned. Thus the cerebellar and brainstem innervations remain intact. If as has been plausibly suggested (Olds 1975), the locus coeruleus system functions as a whole, transmitting the same reinforcement signal to different brain regions, there may well be considerable redundancy, with one set of collaterals substituting for another.

Even with the 6-OH-dopamine lesions confined to the ascending fibres some findings consistent with the hypothesis have been reported. Thus deficits have been found in the acquisition of a light–dark discrimination response (Mason and Iversen 1975) and in a spatial-learning task (Mason and Fibiger 1978). Thus it might be suggested that those situations which furthest extend the rat's learning capacity are those in which deficits following incomplete lesions of the locus coeruleus system can be demonstrated. Furthermore in those relatively simple situations (e.g. acquisition of a bar-pressing response with continuous reinforcement), in which dorsal bundle lesions fail to affect acquisition, there are deficits in extinction and these deficits depend on the lesion being present during acquisition (Mason and Fibiger 1978). This is shown by the finding that the changes in extinction do not occur if the lesions are made after learning.

The situation concerning the role of noradrenalin in learning can be summarized as follows:

1. Pharmacological experiments (e.g. with diethyldithiocarbamate and intraventricular noradrenalin) rather strongly support the view that central noradrenergic neurons are involved in establishing the memory trace.

2. While some experiments with electrolytic lesions of the locus coeruleus have yielded results consistent with the hypothesis that this is the reinforcement system (as originally suggested by electrical self-stimulation experiments; Crow *et al*. 1972), the findings with 6-OH-dopamine have been difficult to interpret. Most have been thought to refute the hypothesis, but some effects on acquisition are apparent and the possibility remains that with its multiple collaterals the system maintains a high level of redundancy.

Some recent experiments with the neurotoxin DSP-4 which, being administered peripherally may cause more extensive degenerations of central noradrenergic terminals, have shown apparent impairments of acquisition of an active-avoidance response (Ogren *et al.* 1981).

Thus the hypothesis that the coerulocortical noradrenergic system is involved in converting short- to long-term memory traces has yet to be decisively refuted. Some other theories, e.g. that it mediates anxiety, have been tested and found wanting (Crow *et al.* 1978).

Noradrenalin and dementia

Although cholinergic deficits have been the major focus of interest in Alzheimer's disease, there is now evidence of a loss of noradrenergic neurons. Thus noradrenaline concentrations have been reported to be somewhat reduced in some cases in post-mortem brain (Adolfsson *et al.* 1979), and there were indications from histochemical observations of a loss of noradrenalin-containing terminals in biopsy specimens (Berger *et al.* 1976). Dopamine-β-hydroxylase is a marker enzyme of noradrenergic neurons, and in a post-mortem investigation the activity of this enzyme was reduced in cases of AD (Cross *et al.* 1980; Fig. 3.4).

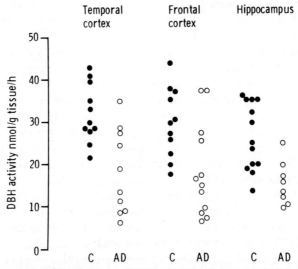

Fig. 3.4. Dopamine-β-hydroxylase (DBH) activity in post-mortem brain tissue of controls (●) and patients with senile dementia of the Alzheimer-type (○).

There is also considerable evidence of a loss of locus coeruleus neurons in dementia (Bondareff *et al.* 1981; Forno 1978; Mann *et al.* 1980; Tomlinson *et al.* 1981). Recent studies of methoxyhydroxy phenylethylene glycol (MHPG) suggest this noradrenalin metabolite may also be decreased in cortical regions in dementia (Cross and Crow, unpublished observations). A study relating the degree of cholinergic and noradrenergic loss to the severity of the disease process, suggests that whereas the cholinergic deficit may be primarily involved, the noradrenergic loss may be a later consequence of the disease (Perry *et al.* 1981).

Patients with Korsakow's psychosis have been found to have reduced concentrations of the noradrenalin metabolite MHPG in cerebrospinal fluid, by

TABLE 3.5

	Korsakoff's syndrome	Controls
HVA	35 ± 6	28 ± 3
5-HIAA	24 ± 6	24 ± 2
VMA	0.6 ± 0.1	1.0 ± 0.2
MHPG	6.1 ± 0.7	*12.1 ± 1.1

$*p < 0.01$.
From McEntee and Mair (1978).

comparison with controls (McEntee and Mair 1978; Table 3.5). Within this patient group, reduced MHPG was highly correlated with memory impairment.

Thus in both the Korsakow psychosis and in AD there is evidence for a loss of noradrenergic neurons. While in the former condition a significant association between noradrenergic deficits and memory impairment has been reported (McEntee and Mair 1978), in the latter case this remains to be investigated.

CONCLUSIONS

A cholinergic link is involved in the transition from short-term (or primary) to long-term (or secondary) memory. Deficits in memory processes similar to those seen in patients with the amnesic syndrome (Baddeley and Warrington 1970), are seen following administration of centrally-acting cholinergic antagonists. It seems probable that the memory failure which is observed in Alzheimer type dementia is a consequence of loss of cholinergic neurons. That this may be caused by a slow virus is supported by observations that similar neuropathological and neurochemical changes are seen in scrapie.

Some animal experiments suggest the locus coeruleus noradrenergic system also plays a role in learning. The recent finding of reduced concentrations of the noradrenalin metabolite MHPG in cerebrospinal fluid in patients with Korsakoff's psychosis, is consistent with such a relationship. The noradrenergic deficits which are now well-established in Alzheimer-type dementia are probably less directly associated than cholinergic losses with the primary pathological process.

REFERENCES

Adolfsson, R., Gottfried, C. G., Roos, B. E., and Winblad, B. (1979). Changes in the brain catecholamines in patients with dementia of the Alzheimer type. *Br. J. Psychiat.* **135**, 216–33.

Amaral, D. G. and Foss, J. A. (1975). Locus coeruleus lesions and learning. *Science, NY* **88**, 377–8.

Anlezark, G. M., Crow, T. J., and Greenway, A. P. (1973). Impaired learning and decreased cortical norepinephrine after bilateral locus coeruleus lesions. *Science, NY* **181**, 682–4.

Baddeley, A. D. and Warrington, E. K. (1970). Amnesia and the distinction between long- and short-term memory. *J. Verb. Learn. Behav.* **9**, 176–89.

Berger, B., Escourolle, R., and Moyne, M. A. (1976). Axones catecholaminergiques du cortex cerebral humain. *Revue neurol.* **132**, 183–94.

34   *Central neurotransmitters, memory, and dementia*

Bondareff, W., Mountjoy, C. Q., and Roth, M. (1981). Selective loss of neurones of origin of adrenergic projection to cerebral cortex (nucleus locus coeruleus) in senile dementia. *Lancet* i, 783–4.

Bowen, D. M., Smith, C. B., White, P., and Davison, A. N. (1976). Neurotransmitter-related enzymes and indices of hypoxia in senile dementia and other abiotrophies. *Brain* **99**, 459–95.

— White, P., Spillane, J. A., Goodhardt, M J., Curzon, G., Iwangoff, P., Meier-Ruge, W., and Davison, A. N. (1979). Accelerated ageing or selective neuronal loss as an important cause of dementia? *Lancet* i, 11–14.

Crow, T. J. (1968). Cortical synapses and reinforcement: a hypothesis. *Nature, Lond.* **219**, 736–7.

— (1977). A general catecholamine hypothesis. *Neurosci. Res. Progr. Bull.* **15**, 195–205.

— Deakin, J. F. W., File, S. E., Longden, A., and Wandlandt, S. (1978). The locus coeruleus noradrenergic system – evidence against a role in attention, habituation, anxiety and motor activity. *Brain Res.* **155**, 249–62.

— and Grove-White, I. G. (1973). An analysis of the learning deficit following hyoscine administration to man. *Br. J. Pharmac.* **49**, 322–7.

— — and Ross, D. G. (1976). The specificity of the action of hyoscine on human learning. *Br. J. clin. Pharmac.* **2**, 367–8P.

— Spear, P. J., and Arbuthnott, G. W. (1972). Intracranial self-stimulation with electrodes in the region of the locus coeruleus. *Brain Res.* **36**, 275–87.

Davies, P. (1979). Neurotransmitter-related enzymes in senile dementia of Alzheimer type. *Brain Res.* **171**, 319–27.

— and Feisullin, S. (1981). Post-mortem stability of α-bungarotoxin binding sites in mouse and human brain. *Brain Res.* **216**, 449–54.

— and Maloney, A. J. F. (1976). Selective loss of central cholinergic neurons in Alzheimer's disease. *Lancet* ii, 1403.

— and Verth, A. M. (1978). Regional distribution of muscarinic acetylcholine receptor in normal and Alzheimer type dementia brains. *Brain Res.* **138**, 385–92.

Drachman, D. A. and Leavitt, J. (1974). Human memory and the cholinergic system. A relationship to ageing? *Archs Neurol.* **30**, 113–21.

Forno, L. S. (1978). The locus coeruleus in Alzheimers disease. *J. Neuropath. exp. Neurol.* **37**, 614.

Gauss, C. J. (1906). Geburten in Künstlichem Dämmerschlaf. *Arch. Gynaek.* **78**, 579–631.

Ghoneim, M. M. and Mewalt, S. P. (1975). Effects of diazepam and scopolamine on storage, retrieval and organisational processes in memory. *Psychopharmacologia* **44**, 257–62.

Glanzer, M. and Cunitz, A. R. (1966). Two storage mechanisms in free recall. *J. verb. Learn. verb. Behav.* **5**, 351–60.

Hardy, T. K. and Wakely, D. (1962). The amnesic properties of hyoscine and atropine in pre-anaesthetic medication. *Anaesthesia* **17**, 331–6.

Howard, J. L. and Breese, G. R. (1974). Physiological and behavioural effects of centrally-administered 6-hydroxydopamine in cats. *Pharmac. Biochem. Behav.* **2**, 651–61.

Kety, S. S. (1970). The biogenic amines in the central nervous system: their possible roles in arousal, emotion and learning. In *Neurosciences second study program* (ed. F. O. Schmitt) pp. 324–36. Rockefeller University Press, New York.

Koob, G. F., Kelley, A. F., and Mason, S. T. (1978). Locus coeruleus lesions: learning and extinction. *Physiol. Behav.* **20**, 709–16.

Longo, V.G. (1966). Behavioural and electroencephalographic effects of atropine and related compounds. *Pharmac. Rev.* **18**, 965–96.

McDermott, J. R., Fraser, H., and Dickinson, A. G. (1978). Reduced choline acetyltransferase activity in scrapie mouse brain. *Lancet* **ii**, 318–19.
McEntee, W. J. and Mair, R. G. (1978). Memory impairment in Korsakoff's psychosis: a correlation with brain noradrenergic activity. *Science, NY* **202**, 905–7.
Mann, D. M. A., Lincoln, A. J., Yates, P. O., Stamp, J. E., and Toper, S. (1980). Changes in the monoamine containing neurones of the human central nerous system in senile dementia. *Br. J. Psychiat.* **136**, 533–41.
Mason, S. T. and Fibiger, H. C. (1978). Noradrenaline and spatial memory. *Brain Res.* **156**, 382–6.
—— —— (1979). The dorsal bundle extinction effect – dependence on subtle changes in acquision. *Brain Res.* **166**, 341–8.
—— and Iversen, S. D. (1974). Learning impairment in rats after 6-hydroxy-dopamine-induced depletion of brain catecholamines. *Nature, Lond.* **258**, 697–8.
—— —— (1975). Learning in the absence of forebrain noradrenaline. *Nature, Lond.* **258**, 422–4.
Mirsky, A. F. and Kornetsky, C. (1964). On the dissimilar effects of drugs on the digit symbol substitution and continuous performance tests. *Psychopharmacologia* **5**, 161–77.
Ogren, S. O., Archer, T., and Ross, S. B. (1980). Evidence for a role of the locus coeruleus NA system in learning. *Neurosci. Lett.* **20**, 351–6.
Olds, J. (1976). Reward and drive neurons. In *Brain stimulation reward* (ed. A. Wauquier and E. T. Rolls) pp. 1–27. North-Holland, Amsterdam.
Pandit, S. K. amd Dundee, J. W. (1970). Pre-operative amnesia. *Anaesthesia* **25**, 493–9.
—— —— and Keilty, S. R. (1971). Amnesia studies with intravenous medication. *Anaesthesia* **26**, 421–8.
Perry, E. K., Perry, R. H., Blessed, G., and Tomlinson, B. E. (1977). Necropsy evidence of central cholinergic deficits in senile dementia. *Lancet* **i**, 189.
—— Tomlinson, B. E., Blessed, G., Bergmann, K., Gibson, P. H., and Perry, R. H. (1978). Correlation' of cholinergic abnormalities with senile plaques and mental tests scores in senile dementia. *Br. med. J.* **ii**, 1457–9.
—— —— —— Cross, A. J., and Crow, T. J. (1981). Neuropathological and biochemical observations on the noradrenergic system in Alzheimer's disease. *J. neurol. Sci.* **51**, 279–81.
Petersen, R. C. (1977). Scopolamine induced learning failures in man. *Psychopharmacology* **52**, 283–9.
Rainbow, T. C., Adler, J. E., and Flexner, L. B. (1976). Comparison in mice of the amnestic effects of cycloheximide and 6-hydroxydopamine in a one-trial passive avoidance task. *Pharmac. Biochem. Behav.* **4**, 347–9.
Randt, C. T., Quartermain, D., Goldstein, M., and Anagnoste, B. (1971). Norepinephrine biosynthesis inhibition: effects on memory in mice. *Science, NY* **172**, 498–9.
Roberts, D. C. S., Price, M. T. C., and Fibiger, H. C. (1976). The dorsal tegmental noradrenergic projection: an analysis of its role in maze learning. *J. comp. physiol. Psychol.* **90**, 363–72.
Safer, D. J. and Allen, R. P. (1971). The central effects of scopolamine in man. *Biol. Psychiat.* **3**, 347–55.
Sessions, G. R., Kant, G. J., and Koob, G. F. (1976). Locus coeruleus lesions and learning in the rat. *Physiol. Behav.* **17**, 853–9.
Stein, L., Belluzzi, J. D., and Wise, C. D. (1975). Memory enhancement by central administration of norepinephrine. *Brain Res.* **84**, 329–35.
Tomlinson, B. E., Irving, D., and Blessed, G. (1981). Cell loss in the locus coeruleus in senile dementia of the Alzheimer type. *J. neurol. Sci.* **47**, 419–28.

Ungerstedt, U. (1971). Stereotaxic mapping of the monoamine pathways in the rat brain. *Acta physiol. scand.* **367** Suppl., 1–48.
White, P., Hiley, C. R., Goodhardt, M. J., Carrasco, L. H., Keet, J. R., Williams, I. E. I., and Bowen, D. M. (1977). Neocortical cholinergic neurones in elderly people. *Lancet* i, 668–70.
Wisniewski, H. M., Bruce, M. E., and Fraser, H. (1975). Infectious etiology of neuritic (senile) plaques in mice. *Science, NY* **190**, 1108–10.

4

The senile brain

DAVID JOLLEY

Old people are no longer rarities. Better sanitation, cleaner air, and a more reliable supply of food, purchased by industrial wealth, have freed infancy and middle age from the fear of death by infection. The hazards that remain or are gaining significance in these age groups are traceable in many instances to selfish, inconsiderate behaviour, that harms the self or others by violence, excess of food, stimulant drugs or chemicals, often in conjunction with the internal combustion engine or gun. The senium, in contrast is still bestrewn with the same dangers that characterized it for previous generations. Indeed it may be a more perilous experience to be old now than it was in the past (McKeown 1976).

Whilst more people survive into old age, more carry with them disabilities produced by partially-resolved pathologies that arose earlier in life. Even those illnesses that appear in old age are less likely to terminate life, for life expectation within the senium has been increased and more particularly life with disability has been increased here as it has for the young handicapped (Gruenberg and Hagnell 1978). Thus, whilst old people have become common and, therefore, lost the advantages that accrued to the precious patriarch or matriarch, disabled old people have increased in number out of proportion, and are easily viewed *en masse* as an unwelcomed and undesired burden on the rest of post-industrial society.

Sometimes the population statistics, presented to reflect the grown and growing importance of the elderly, become hypnotic and themselves become the focus of preoccupation. Yet each individual old person is fascinatingly unique: a product of inheritance passed through forty million minutes of history and personal experiences, successes and failures, griefs and ecstasy, gains and losses, as well as illnesses of various sorts and dimensions. Involvement with elderly patients is tremendously challenging and interesting, as the relevance of particular themes and incidents in an individual life are traced to solve the puzzle of the moment. This complexity is too much for the research worker, keen to tease out mechanisms relevant to one of the several age-related disorders that may be present in one old person. Thus a good deal of research into the illnesses that are common in old age has used presenile probands who present one such illness at a time.

PSYCHIATRIC DISORDERS IN THE ELDERLY

It was a major step forward when it became clearly recognized that aging itself does not carry with it the inevitability of mental decline, and those old people who demonstrate changes in mood, perception, personality, and/or cognition, are suffering from pathological states of mind which can be approached with the same tools and similar expectations to those found in younger people (Bromley 1974).

Old people are at least as prone to psychiatric disorders as younger people and present a range of symptoms including anxiety, fear, obsessions, hypochondriasis, and depression of varying quality and severity, as well as hypomania and persecutory states (Pitt 1974). These will be considered in detail in later chapters in this book. Yet the most characteristic mental disorders of the senium are the confusional states and dementing syndromes of organic brain impairment (Jolley 1981a; Jolley and Arie 1980). For while mood disorders are numerically more common than organic psychosyndromes, it is these latter that dominate our thinking, both professional and personal, toward mental and emotional life in old age. The greatest fear of the middle aged is not the prospect of physical infirmity, nor boredom, nor depression, these seem tangible and could be coped with by an appropriate strategy. It is the fear of 'becoming senile' − simple, unable to comprehend the world about them, nor to fend for the self. A return to primitive and child-like ways of thinking, behaving, and coping, but only by courtesy of others. This fear explains much of the alienation experienced by many elderly people and the repulsion felt toward them by the young, who seek solace in denial that there is a continuity between 'me' − young and able minded, and 'them' − unable to converse on equal nor even limited terms.

Confused old people have been recognized as such for generations and have needed a lot of care. By and large they have received it and continue to receive it − from their families, welfare agencies, and medical and nursing agencies (Jolley 1981b). Studies based upon careful clinical observations have led us out of the chaos and gloom of the portmanteau diagnosis 'senile psychosis'; the mood disorders and paranoid states have been dissected clear and can now receive extremely useful treatment (Roth and Morrissey 1952; Post 1962, 1966). What remain are the related but distinguishable acute, subacute, and chronic organic brain syndromes: 'delirium' or 'confusional states' and dementing syndromes.

PATTERNS OF CARE

It is undeniable that many old people designated 'confused' or 'senile' by those who care for them, can be helped by modern medical practice. Yet this does not mean that medicine is pre-eminent in the provision of help − much more is achieved by established patterns of familial or local care and acceptance. The essence of the clinican's burden is to be available and to make available all those facilities of modern medical know-how, that will elucidate an understanding and treatment of treatable components of impaired cerebral function, without weakening nor undermining the position of his patient in the community, and, where necessary, to enhance it by encouraging extra supports (Arie 1970). In the present balance of care 94 per cent of 'old people' live in private households, if the sixty-fifth birthday is used to delineate 'old age'. Yet most 65 year olds have another decade to run before they acquire the true stigma of 'senility' − vulnerability and dependence.

Dementia is found in only 4 per cent of 65 year olds, 25 per cent of 75 year olds and up to 60 per cent of 80 year olds (Nielsen 1963). The likelihood of surviving and finding acceptance in the community when suffering from dementia, is related to social circumstances and established personality, more than the severity of impairment. Thus very few dements survive alone for any length of time (Kay *et al.* 1970). An elderly spouse, even though also infirm, is frequently the most robust and enduring supporter. An unmarried daughter or brother or sister may make do and amends, but married daughters, sons, and daughters-in-law have too many other interests, responsibilities, and higher expectations of life, to fall servant to the simple, persistent needs of a dementing relative. A peace-loving grateful soul is more likely to secure neighbourly attention than an irritable, hostile, hypochondriacal, or miserable body.

Help in the house

Many resources are directed to helping relatives maintain dements at home, so that district nurses, home helps, and 'meals-on-wheels' find their way into these homes. Even so demented people make considerable use of the few institutional beds that are available and though they constitute only 5–10 per cent of the old-age population, they contribute at least 50 per cent of the 6 per cent that are housed in hospitals and residential homes. Managing groups of elderly people containing high concentrations of confused individuals, is not easy and puts demands upon the physical attributes of the institution: for safety, availability of toilet and bathing facilities, as well as warmth and shelter. In addition staff require unusual qualities of patience, sympathy and good humour, and consider-able skill in engineering the social environment, so that it is stimulating and reassuring without provoking distress or inducing apathy. Co-residents who are not confused sometimes complain bitterly of exposure to irritating, unrewarding, and, occasionally, frightening behaviour. Visitors, be they relatives, volunteers, or professionals, may find it difficult to tolerate the limited and often simple and crude quality of life that is optimal for the more disabled dements (Evans *et al.* 1980). Expensive and unfashionable as it is, continuing care for people with dementia is hard to establish, let alone maintain, in a position at the centre of the nation's thinking, although it can be cogently argued that this is the most characterstic need of our present society.

DEMENTIA IN OLD AGE

What of dementia in old age? Is this still a useful and appropriate term, or should it be replaced by a modern alternative or euphemism? It may be helpful to draw an analogy with the usage of another 'difficult' and equally important word: 'cancer' is a term well used in fund-raising projects but hastily avoided in a clinical setting. Thus medical students are taught to shuffle the cards from 'carcinoma' to 'mitotic lesion' in order to obscure their discussion from the patient's understanding so that he or she is protected from the fear and helpless-ness engendered by lay beliefs associated with cancer. 'Dementia' is sometimes avoided as a descriptive term for it too may induce fear and trepidation in the sufferer and her relatives and therapeutic nihilism in the responsible doctor. Yet one of the currently more respected but delimited synonyms 'Alzheimer's disease' was presented on a recent television programme as 'a sinister, killing illness' – hardly likely to calm an anxious brow. Surely the terror and infamy of 'dementia' should be capitalized upon for raising funds for research and better services. Alternative terms may be useful in obfuscating discussion for the benefit of patients so long as they do not do the same for the professionals.

As a syndrome

Used in the way that Lishman has detailed (Lishman 1978), dementia as a syndrome characterized by 'acquired global impairment of memory or personality but without impairment of consciousness' is well recognized, time honoured, and avoids the uncertainties and inconsistencies that may befall alternative terminologies. As a syndrome it has a number of possible aetiologies and a range of prognoses (Stout and Jolley 1981). In the elderly it is usual for a number of factors to contribute to the dementing syndrome presented in an individual patient, and though some factors are currently irreversible, others can at least be understood and sometimes manipulated to improve the quality and experience of life for the patient and those who care for him or her.

As an illness

Clinical practice devines that most elderly patients presenting with a dementing syndrome are suffering from one of the two progressive dementing illnesses: senile dementia, which is now usually described as Alzheimer type (SDAT), or arteriosclerotic (multiple-infarct) dementia. Corsellis (1962) demonstrated that even the much maligned acumen of mental hospital psychiatrists, reflected by their equally maligned routine notes, bore a very close relationship to pathological findings of these two major dementing illnesses. At the present time, despite the emergence of powerful new tools that have facilitated investigation and understanding of brain structure, function, and biochemistry in these conditions, neither is amenable to prevention or treatment (Jolley and Arie, 1980).

CONTRIBUTING FACTORS

Physical

There may be other physical factors contributing to the impaired cerebral function, some of which act directly, as for example, intracranial and systemic conditions.

Intracranial conditions:

Space-occupying lesions	Vascular abnormalities
Trauma	Epilepsy
Infarctions	

Systemic conditions:

Infections	Endocrine disorders
Vascular problems	Vitamin deficiencies
Anoxia	Pharmacy; especially polypharmacy
Metabolic disorders	Alcohol

Other factors act indirectly by producing discomfort and overarousal, or as a result of reduced sensory input:

Discomfort	Sensory input
Pain	Poor hearing
Constipation	Poor eyesight
Incontinence	Immobility
	Weightlessness

Emotional

In addition, emotional and other mental disorders may be operative in reducing cerebral performance. Among these, states of depression with or without anxiety, agitation, obsessional, or hypochondriacal features are most important. They impair concentration, decision making and communication and may in themselves produce a pseudodementing picture. Indeed it is interesting that severe depressive states in the elderly produce some neurophysiological changes, e.g. in barbiturate tolerance, that are similar to those associated with the dementing illnesses (Cawley *et al*. 1973).

Environmental

Factors in the social environment are often important, but should not be misrepresented. There is no reliable evidence to support the notion that poverty or social disadvantage are causative of either of the major dementing illnesses. It is, however, undeniable that under-stimulating or suffocating living situations reduce cerebral performance by boredom-induced torpor. Conversely excessive stress can occur when an old person just cannot cope alone and is overcome by helplessness — or is placed alongside very noisy or boisterous youngsters — such situations may push that individual beyond an optimal level of arousal and confound all efforts at mentation.

CONFUSIONAL STATES

Acute or subacute delirious states, confusional states (Lipowski 1980) present more florid symptomatology than the dementias and include variability in the level of consciousness. They are frequently underwritten by one of the dementing illnesses in the elderly and the range of aetiologies is broadly similar to that outlined for the dementia syndrome. The major difference is in the speed of development of pathological processes rather than in their nature.

THERAPEUTIC POSSIBILITIES (Fig. 4.1)

Faced with a dementing syndrome or confusional state in an old person, the clinician finds much to tax his diagnostic abilities and the challenging likelihood that a good deal can be offered to help a situation, by controlling, reversing, or alleviating these contributory factors.

Underlying organic disorders

Identification of physical pathology contributing to the syndrome raises the

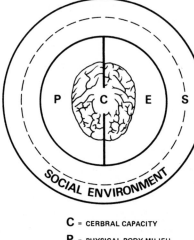

C = CERBRAL CAPACITY
P = PHYSICAL BODY MILIEU
E = EMOTIONAL SET
S = QUALITY OF SENSORY INPUT

Fig. 4.1. Model of levels of function with potential for contributing to dementia.

possibility of treating the 'heart of the matter'. A subdural haematoma may be drained, an intracranial tumour removed, infections, be they local or systemic, are often treatable with antibiotics. Anoxia may be obviated by the use of supplemented supply of the gas and/or by treating the respiratory failure, cardiac insufficiency, or whatever lies at its base. Metabolic disorders and endocrine disorders can be corrected by supplements of missing elements and removal of poisonous accumulations, whilst vitamin deficiencies can be made good. The effects of drugs, be they self- or physician-administered, can often be avoided simply by stopping the offending agent and using an alternative, or indeed nothing at all.

Similarly pain and discomfort attributable to physical problems can usually be alleviated by careful attention. Bowels can be evacuated and then regulated. Urinary incontinence can be sometimes avoided and, more often, rendered less messy and embarrassing by the use of appropriate aids. Suitable analgesia or efficient splinting assuages the pain of shingles or a broken limb, and chiropody may render feet less hostile members of the body.

Removing those factors that may be positively impairing cerebral function is one thing. Yet equally important is the exercise of accepting that some impairment is present, but taking care to give the remaining abilities the best possible chance of functioning well. Poor hearing may be improved by as simple a manoeuvre as removing wax, or else the renewal of an exhausted hearing-aid battery. Visual impairment may be removed, when caused by cataract, by ophthalmic surgery, or clean appropriate spectacles may be of help.

The emotional component

Anxiety, depression, or paranoid thinking respond to treatment with anxiolytics, antidepressants, and neuroleptic medication respectively, in a dementing brain as they do in an organically-preserved brain. It is true there may be difficulties in using them: unwanted effects are common and the margin between therapeutic and toxic regimes is narrowed by increased and often variable end-organ sensitivity. Yet these difficulties can be overcome in many instances and an agitated, disturbed, deranged old man can be transformed to a calm, forgetful, but manageable one.

Manipulating the environment

In all these interventions the physician can see a role. Yet they are as if nothing if confounded by a hostile or unsympathetic social environment. The significance of maintaining demented people in their own homes has been mentioned, together with the importance of acceptable and accepting caring individuals, among whom elderly husbands and wives reign supreme. In addition professionals: nurses, occupational therapists, psychologists, even educationalists, have begun to explore the possibilities of manipulating the personal and group environments of demeted people, to achieve therapeutic effects (Jolley 1979). Here there is no claim to change the dementing process 'at root' — much as may be achieved for instance by removing an unsuspected chronic haematoma. The aim is rather to mould the environment to become, as Albert Kushlick has so helpfully put it, 'a prosthesis'. In this they are extrapolating from the principles inately understood by the husband who takes his wife shopping with him — but himself makes all the decisions on what to buy. When they return to the kitchen he has in mind what meal to produce, when, and how. But he allows and encourages her to be part of the activity, by being in the kitchen, talking about the food, and in his directions to her as to which items to peel. Yet, he is sure that he switches the heat on at the appropriate time, checks the correct temperature is attained and so on. By these means he erects an energizing flexible 'prosthesis', that is reprogrammed minute by minute to take account of changing circumstances.

Prosthetic tools

Despite some notable initiatives in the field of social or environmental therapy, it seems to me that there is likely to be much greater potential in the idea of making good the defects produced by dementia by prosthetic tools. At present these are generally people-based. This is nice and I do not see any lessening of need for personal involvement in caring for confused old people. Yet electronic surveillance and cuing devices have become very sophisticated yet relatively cheap. Most department stores use markers, television cameras, and other equipment to seek and find thieves. We have seen men flown to and from the moon, and spacecraft send back detailed pictures of far-distant planets. If similar resources were directed to refining equipment to cue demented people with information they cannot generate for themselves, I doubt the electronics industry would be found impotent.

FUTURE AIMS

Startling strides have been made in our understanding of the histopathology, neurophysiology, and biochemistry of the elderly brain, devastated by what we believe to be dementing illnesses. These are discussed in greater detail in the ensuing chapters of this volume and these advances hold up some hope of attacking dementia at its very heart. Such an approach is exciting and aesthetically appealing. Yet it is a huge jump to make, from the position that these new pieces of knowledge have made possible, to effectively treating and managing dementia in old people.

In practice there are usually many factors that have come together to impair an elderly brain. There are, therefore, several avenues for therapeutic potential and research endeavour. Some are currently being explored with great vigour, whilst others are relatively neglected. I believe that if we take this problem more seriously, explore these other avenues with greater energy and seek to draw in the expertise of other disciplines, we have the possibility of achieving a much greater and more useful impact on the lives of demented people than has been realized.

REFERENCES

Arie, T. (1970). The first year of the Goodmayes Psychiatric Services for old people. *Lancet* ii, 1179–82.
Bromley, D. (1974). *The psychology of human ageing*. Penguin, Harmondsworth, Middlesex.
Cawley, R. H., Post, F., and Whitehead, A. (1973). Barbiturate tolerance and psychological functioning in elderly depressed patients. *Psychol. Med.* 3, 39–52.
Corsellis, J. (1962). *Mental illness and the ageing brain*. Maudsley Monograph No. 9. Oxford University Press, London.
Evans, G., Hughes, B., and Wilkin, D. [with Jolley, D.] (1980). The management of mental and physical impairment in non-specialist residential homes for the elderly. University Hospital of South Manchester, Psychogeriatric Unit. Research Report No. 4.
Gruenberg, E. M. (1978). Epidemiology of senile dementia. *Adv. Neurol.* 19, 437–57.
Jolley, D. (1979). All is not lost. In *New methods of mental health care* (ed. M. Meacher). Mental Health Foundation, London; Pergamon Press, Oxford.
— (1981a). Acute confusional states in the elderly. In *Acute geriatric medicine* (ed. D. Coakley). Croom Helm, London.
— (1981b). Dementia: misfits in need of care. In *Health care of the elderly* (ed. T. Arie). Croom Helm, London.
— and Arie, T. (1980). Dementia in old age: an outline of current issues. *Hlth Trends* 12, 1–4.
Kay, D. W. K., Bergmann, K., Foster, E. M., McKechnie, A. A., and Roth, M. (1970). Mental illness and hospital usage in the elderly. *Comp. Psychiat.* 1, 26–35.
Lipowski, Z. J. (1980). Delirium updated. *Comp. Psychiat.* 21, 190–6.
Lishman, W. A. (1978). *Organic psychiatry*. Blackwell, Oxford.
McKeown, T. (1976). *The modern rise of population*. Edward Arnold, London.
Nielson, J. (1963). Geronto-psychiatric period prevalence investigation in a geographically delimited population. *Acta psychiat. scand.* 38, 307–30.
Pitt, B. (1974). *Psychogeriatrics*. Churchill Livingstone, Edinburgh.
Post. F. (1962). *The significance of affective symptoms in old age*. Maudsley Monograph. Oxford University Press, London.
— (1966). *Persistent persecutory states of the elderly*. Pergamon Press, Oxford.

Roth, M. and Morrissey, D. (1952). Problems in the diagnosis and classification of mental disorder in old age. *J. Ment. Sci.* **93**, 66–72.
Stout, I. and Jolley, D. (1981). The dementia syndrome and how to recognise it. *Geriat. Med.* February, 15–18.

5

The pharmokinetics of psychotropic drugs in the elderly

ROBIN BRAITHWAITE

INTRODUCTION

There is general clinical agreement that the elderly are both more sensitive to drugs and suffer from an increased incidence of adverse reactions compared with younger patients. Thus, in one study reported by Seidl *et al.* (1966), 24 per cent of those patients aged over 80 years had adverse drug reactions, compared with only 12 per cent in patients aged 41 –50 years. In an extensive study carried out by Hurwitz (1969) in Belfast on more than 1000 in-patients, the overall rate of adverse drug reactions was 10 per cent compared with a rate of 15 per cent in patients aged over 60 and 20 per cent in patients over 70 years. Studies carried out in out-patients have also shown a similar picture (Learoyd 1972; Caranasos *et al.* 1974). Of particular significance is the study by Learoyd (1972) who reported that of 236 consecutive admissions to a psychogeriatric unit, 16 per cent were due to adverse reactions to psychotropic drugs. Moreover, many patients improved when their medication was either stopped or the dose reduced. This increased incidence of adverse reactions to drugs may partly be due to the fact that the elderly suffer from more disease and receive more drugs than younger patients.

ROLE OF PHARMACOKINETICS

An apparent increase in drug sensitivity may be due to an impairment in drug handling, so-called pharmacokinetic changes, and/or changes in the number or sensitivity of drug-receptor sites, so-called pharmacodynamic changes. There is good evidence that both types of modification take place as part of the aging process. However, for the purpose of this presentation I will devote most of my attention to pharmacokinetic changes in the elderly.

The role of pharmacokinetics is to provide a mathematical basis for the description and prediction of the time course of drugs and their metabolites in the body. A schematic representation of the major pharmacokinetic events following drug administration is shown in Fig. 5.1. It is the interindividual variation in these different parameters which determines the concentration of drug at the receptor site. There are a number of physiological changes which take place with aging, which are capable of modifying certain pharmacokinetic parameters in a particular way. The most important of these changes along with their pharmacokinetic consequences are summarized in Table 5.1.

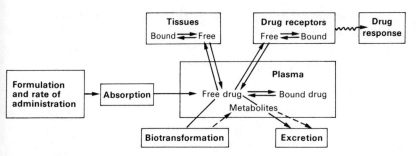

Fig. 5.1 Simplified scheme of pharmacokinetics.

TABLE 5.1. *Influence of physiological changes on pharmacokinetics in the elderly. (Modifed from Vestal (1978).)*

Effect	Altered physiological function	Action
Absorption	↑ Gastric pH	No consistent change reported
	↓ Gastric blood-flow	
	↓ Gut motility	
Distribution	↓ Body weight (particularly very old)	↑ Dose per unit body weight
		Water-soluble drugs:
	↓ Lean body mass	↑ Blood levels
	↑ Adipose tissue	↓ Distribution volume
	↓ Total body water	*Lipid-soluble drugs:*
		↓ Blood levels
		↑ Distribution volume
	↓ Plasma albumin	↓ Plasma binding ↑ free fraction
	↑ Plasma α_1-acid glycoprotein	↑ Plasma binding ↓ free fraction
Elimination Renal	↓ GFR	↓ Excretion of water soluble drugs and metabolites
	↓ Tubular secretion	
	↓ Renal blood flow	
Hepatic	↓ Hepatic mass	↓ Clearance
	↓ Liver blood-flow	↑ First-pass availability of some drugs
	↓ Enzyme activity	

DRUG ABSORPTION

There are several physiological changes which might at first sight be expected to influence drug absorption (Bender 1968; Stevenson *et al.* 1979). These are: decrease in gastric output with subsequent increase in gastric pH, reductions in splanchnic blood-flow, gut motility, and the rate of gastric emptying. The absorption of a number of dietary constituents such as galactose, calcium, iron, and thiamine, are known to be reduced in the elderly, but these are all absorbed by active-transport mechanisms. The majority of drugs are, however, absorbed by a process of passive diffusion and would, therefore, not be influenced in the same way (Bender 1968). Although only a relatively small number of drugs has been studied so far, the results indicate that drug absorption in the elderly appears to be unimpaired (Stevenson *et al.* 1979). Although high plasma drug concentrations have sometimes been observed in elderly patients following the oral administration of some drugs, this is probably due to differences in drug distribution or elimination rather than absorption.

Single night-time dosage

Partly as a means of simplifying drug-dosage regimes and improving drug compliance, there has been a recent trend towards the use of single night-time dosage regimes of some drugs, particularly the tricyclic antidepressants. At first sight this would seem reasonable from a certain pharmacokinetic standpoint, in that many of these drugs have elimination half-lives of the order of 24 hours or more. More important considerations are perhaps peak and dosage interval variation in plasma drug concentrations. Figure 5.2 shows the mean (± SEM) plasma amitriptyline concentrations recorded in eight healthy volunteers given a single oral dose of 75 mg amitriptyline, in the form of a standard (Saroten) or sustained release (Lentizol) formulation. The study was carried out according to a randomized balanced design following an overnight fast. Following ingestion of Saroten, recorded peak plasma amitriptyline concentrations ranged between 31 and 59 µg/l (mean 40 µg/l), these being achieved at between 3–4 h after administration. Following ingestion of Lentizol, peak plasma amitriptyline concentrations ranged between 16–41 µg/l (mean 23 µg/l) at between 4–12 hours after administration. The mean plasma amitriptyline elimination half-life (17.9 ± 1.7 h following Saroten and 19.8 ± 3.2 h following Lentizol) was similar to that recorded in other studies.

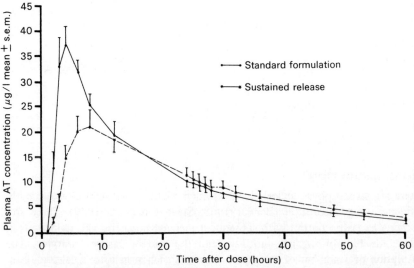

Fig. 5.2. Mean (± SEM) plasma amitriptyline concentrations in eight subjects following a single oral dose (75 mg) of two different formulations of amitriptyline.

The bioavailability of the two formulations, as judged by AUC values at 60 hours and infinity were not significantly different. The mean plasma drug concentration data obtained in these subjects was used to simulate plasma drug concentrations that would be achieved on repeated dosing. The variation in dosage-interval plasma amitriptyline concentrations on a single (75 mg) night-time dosage regime, were considerably greater using the ordinary formulation although mean steady-state levels were the same. It is likely that the higher peak plasma amitriptyline concentrations obtained following repeated night-time medication with a standard formulation, will produce a greater incidence of side-effects, as compared with the same dose of sustained release formulation. This can be particularly important in the elderly, where side-effects to tricyclic antidepressant therapy are a more serious problem.

DRUG DISTRIBUTION

Body composition undergoes a number of important changes with the aging process which can have a marked influence on drug distribution. The elderly tend to weigh less than younger patients, particularly the very old, and the use of standard dosage regimes will, as a consequence, result in generally higher blood and tissue concentrations of drugs. As patients get older, total body water tends to decline, there is also an increase in adipose tissue and a reduction in lean body mass. In a study by Novak (1972), body composition in a group of subjects aged 65–86 years was compared with that obtained in subjects aged 18–25 years. The percentage of body fat increased from 18 to 36 per cent of body weight in males and from 33 to 45 per cent in females. Thus, the result of such changes in body composition may vary according to sex as well as age. The result of changes in body composition will also vary according to the type of drug used. With lipid-soluble drugs, which include most of the psychotropic drugs in common use, there will be a relative distribution of drug into fatty tissues, so that blood and plasma concentrations will tend to be lower and distribution volumes larger. As a direct result of any increase in distribution volume there will be an increase in elimination half-life. In the case of water-soluble or polar compounds the opposite situation will arise, and there will be a trend towards higher blood and plasma concentrations and smaller distribution volumes.

Plasma-protein binding

Another important factor influencing the distribution of drugs is plasma-protein binding. It is the free unbound fraction of drug in plasma that is 'pharmacologi-cally active' and in direct equilibrium with drug-receptor sites (Fig. 5.1). Any alteration in the proportion of drug bound to plasma proteins may, therefore, have important consequences. Although plasma albumin declines with age, the concentration of other plasma proteins may actually increase (Cammarata *et al.* 1967; Woodford-Williams *et al.* 1964). Many psychotropic drugs are highly bound to plasma proteins, but the binding affinity to albumin may be weak. It has recently been shown by Piafsky *et al* (1978) that a number of cationic drugs (including several psychotropic drugs) are strongly bound to an acute-phase reactant protein, α_1-acid glycoprotein, and studies have shown that the plasma concentration of this protein increases as a consequence of various disease states, such as bacterial infection, carcinoma, and inflammatory disease. This can lead to an increase in the plasma-protein binding of those drugs which have a high affinity for this protein. The presence of multiple disease states is very common in the elderly (Vestel 1978) and likely to be associated with increased plasma concentrations of α_1-acid glycoprotein (Braithwaite et al. 1978). The influence of age and the presence of multiple disease states is, therefore, going to lead to a complicated situation with regard to overall changes in plasma protein binding and one where simple predictions cannot be made.

DRUG ELIMINATION

Renal excretion

Glomerular filtration rate (GFR) is reduced in the elderly, there being an average decline in function of some 35 per cent between the ages of 20 and 90 years (Rowe et al. 1976). Also, renal blood-flow, tubular secretion, and urine concentrating ability during water deprivation, all decline with age. It is, therefore, possible to show that there is some impairment in the clearance of water-soluble drugs or metabolites, whose chief route of elimination is via the kidney (Kampmann and Mølholm 1979). Lithium is the best known psychotropic drug to be eliminated through the kidney, and intoxication may be complicated by renal insufficiency. Reduced renal concentrating ability is also a common complication with long-term lithium treatment (Hansen 1981). For these reasons, lithium treatment should be carefully controlled in the elderly.

Hepatic elimination

The vast majority of psychotropic drugs are eliminated from the body by metabolism in the hepatic microsomal enzyme system. In the elderly there are possible reductions in hepatic mass, liver blood-flow, and microsomal enzyme activity, which are all likely to lead to some impairment in the body's ability to metabolize drugs and other foreign compounds (Stevenson et al. 1979). In a number of early studies plasma elimination half-life was used as an index of drug metabolism, but this is misleading since half-life may just as easily be influenced by changes in distribution volume, as by changes in clearance. The most reliable indicator of drug metabolizing capacity is total clearance. A clear indication that the elderly have some impairment in the ability to metabolize drugs has emerged from studies by O'Malley et al. (1971) on antipyrene. It was shown that antipyrene plasma half-life was 50 per cent longer and its clearance 40 per cent reduced, in elderly subjects compared with younger controls. There are now data on a number of other drugs when similar findings have been observed, but the overall picture is far from simple.

Benzodiazepines

The effect of age on the pharmacokinetics of the benzodiazepine groups of drugs has been investigated in more detail than perhaps any other group of compounds. Preliminary studies by Klotz et al. (1975) on diazepam showed that its plasma half-life was prolonged in the elderly and that its distribution volume was also increased. But, there was no significant reduction in plasma clearance. In more detailed studies carried out by Greenblatt *et al.* (1980), the influence of other factors, such as sex, protein binding, and cigarette smoking, were also considered. These studies showed that diazepam half-life was prolonged in both elderly males and females. However, distribution volume was larger in females than males regardless of age, and larger in the elderly regardless of sex. Diazepam plasma-protein binding was also reduced in the elderly, mainly as a consequence of reduced albumin concentrations. The clearance of unbound diazepam tended to be higher in females than in males of both young and old subjects, and was higher in the young than in the elderly of both sexes. Smoking was also associated with higher clearance values. With such a complex situation it is perhaps difficult to generalize to the situation with other benzodiazepines. However, it would seem that for those benzodiazepines which undergo oxidative metabolic trans-formations (e.g. diazepam, chlordiazepoxide, flurazepam, and desmethyl-diazepam), drug half-lives are increased, distribution volumes increase and clearances are reduced (Greenblatt and Shader 1980). For those benzodiazepines which undergo simple glucuronide conjugation (e.g. oxazepam, temazepam and lorazepam), the aging process appears to exert only a minimal influence on drug clearance (Greenblatt and Shader 1980). This can have an important influence on the choice of hypnotic in the elderly.

Tricyclic antidepressants

The tricyclic antidepressants have been less well investigated. Niess *et al.* (1977) reported a significant correlation between age and steady-state plasma concen-trations, of imipramine, desipramine and amitriptyline, but not nortriptyline. Similar results were reported by Braithwaite *et al.* (1979) for amitriptyline and nortriptyline. Niess *et al.* (1977) also reported an increased elimination half-life for desipramine, but not imipramine, in elderly patients, but the significance of these findings is uncertain. A more detailed investigation of the influence of age on the pharmacokinetics of tricyclic antidepressants was carried out by Dawling *et al.* (1980). In this study 20 patients (19 female and 1 male) aged between 68 and 100 years (mean age 81 years) suffering from a variety of physical disorders, but also sufficiently depressed to warrant treatment with a tricyclic antidepressant drug, were given single and repeated doses of nortriptyline. The plasma elimination half-life (Fig. 5.3) and total oral clearance (Fig. 5.4) of nortriptyline in these patients was significantly different from that observed in young healthy volunteers, although there was no direct correlation between age and kinetic parameters in both patients and volunteers.

The patient group differed from the young control group, not only in age and sex distribution, but also because the subjects were hospitalized and suffering from various physical disorders. In many cases patients were suffering from multiple disease states and most patients were also receiving treatment with a wide variety of drugs. For these reasons the differences in nortriptyline pharmaco-kinetics between the two groups was probably only partly due to age differences, and the presence of physical illness and medication may have been a more important factor. Some evidence of this argument may be found in a study reported by Turbott *et al.* (1980). This group investigated the pharmacokinetics

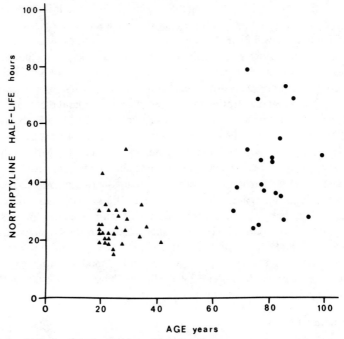

Fig. 5.3. Relationship between age and plasma nortriptyline half-life in elderly patients ($n = 20$) and young healthy volunteers ($n = 30$). (Adapted from Dawling *et al.* (1980) and unpublished material.)

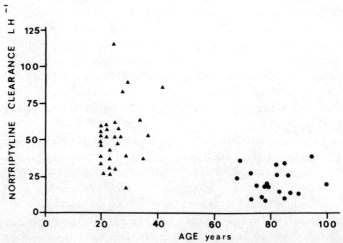

Fig. 5.4. Relationship between age and plasma nortriptyline clearance in elderly patients ($n = 20$) and young healthy volunteers ($n = 30$). (Adapted from Dawling *et al.* (1980) and unpublished material.)

of nortriptyline in a group of 10 healthy volunteers free from medication (age range 66–79 years), and found the values obtained for half-life and clearance to be similar to those reported in younger healthy volunteers.

CONCLUSIONS

It is clear that there is no consistent pattern of change with regard to pharmacokinetics and aging. The disposition of some drugs may be impaired in some elderly patients; which may be the cause of increased drug sensitivity in certain situations. It can be very difficult to separate the relative influence of aging (chronological or biological) and gender, from that of multiple disease states and also environmental factors such as medication, diet, and use of tobacco and alcohol. Thus, in the absence of any simple guide, each drug should be individually investigated using appropriate pharmacokinetic tests. At the same time, it is important not to lose site of the possible importance of pharmacodynamic changes in the elderly (Castelden and George 1979). Homeostasis in general becomes less responsive with age so that the elderly may be more susceptible to drug toxicity than younger patients.

It follows that extra care should be taken with the elderly in the choice of appropriate drug, its formulation and dosage regime. As a general rule the elderly will require smaller doses than are customarily given to younger patients.

Acknowledgements

I should like to thank Mrs Gill Cartwright for her help in the preparation of this manuscript.

REFERENCES

Bender, A. D. (1968). Effect of age on intestinal absorption: implications for drug absorption in the elderly. *J. Am. Geriat. Soc.* **16**, 1331–9.

Braithwaite, R. A., Hard, R., and Snape, A. (1978). Plasma protein binding of maprotiline in geriatric patients – influence of α_1 acid glycoprotein. *Br. J. clin. Pharmac.* **6**, 448–9.

— Montgomery, S., and Dawling, S. (1979). Age, depression and tricyclic antidepressant levels. In *Drugs and the elderly – perspectives in geriatric clinical pharmacology* (ed. J. Crooks and I. H. Stevenson) pp. 133–43. Macmillan, London.

Cammarata, R. J., Rodnan, G. P., and Fennell, R. H. (1967). Serum antigammaglobulin and anti-nuclear factors in the aged. *J. Am. med. Ass.* **199**, 115–18.

Caranasos, G. J., Stewart, R. B., and Cluff, L. E. (1974). Drug induced illness leading to hospitalization. *J. Am. med. Ass.* **228**, 713–17.

Castleden, C. M. and George, C. F. (1979). Increased sensitivity to benzodiazepines in the elderly. In *Drugs and the elderly – perspectives in geriatric clinical pharmacology* (ed. J. Crooks and I. H. Stevenson) pp. 169–78. Macmillan, London.

Dawling, S., Crome, P., and Braithwaite, R. A. (1980). Pharmacokinetics of single oral doses of nortriptyline in depressed elderly hospital patients and young healthy volunteers. *Clin. Pharmacokinet.* **5**, 394–401.

Greenblatt, D. J., Allen, M. D., Harmatz, J. S. and Shader, R. I. (1980). Diazepam disposition determinants. *Clin. Pharmac. Ther.* **27**, 301–12.

— and Shader, R. I. (1980). Effect of age and other drugs on Benzodiazepine kinetics. *Arzneimittel-Forsch.* **30**, 886–90.

Hansen, H. E. (1981). Renal toxocity of lithium. *Drugs* **22**, 461–76.

Hurwitz, N. (1969). Predisposing factors in adverse reactions to drugs. *Br. med. J.* i, 536–40.

Kampmann, J. P. and Mølholm, J. E. (1979). Renal excretion of drugs. In *Drugs and the elderly – perspectives in geriatric clinical pharmacology* (ed. J. Crooks and I. H. Stevenson) pp. 77–87. Macmillan, London.

Klotz, U., Avant, G. R., Hoyumpa, A., Schenker, S., and Wilkinson, G. R. (1975). The effect of age and liver disease on the disposition and elimination of diazepam in adult man. *J. clin. Invest.* **55**, 347–59.

Learoyd, B. M. (1972). Psychotropic drugs and the elderly patient. *Med. J. Aust.* **1**, 1131.

Niess, A., Robinson, D. S., Friedman, M. J., Green, R., Cooper, T. B., Ravaris, C. L., and Ives, J. O. (1977). Relationship between age and tricyclic antidepressant plasma levels. *Am. J. Psychol.* **134**, 790–3.

Novak, L. P. (1972). Aging, total body potassium fat free mass, and cell mass in males and females aged 28–35 years. *J. Geront.* **27**, 438–43.

O'Malley, K., Crooks, J., Duke, E., and Stevenson, I. H. (1971). Effect of age and sex on human drug metabolism. *Br. med. J.* **iii**, 607–9.

Piafsky, K. M., Borgå, O., Odarcederlöf, I., Johansson, C., and Sjoqvist, F. (1978). Increased plasma protein binding of propranolol and chlorpromazine mediated by disease-induced elevations of plasma α_1 acid glycoprotein. *New Engl. J. Med.* **299**, 1435–9.

Rowe, J. W., Andres, R., Tobin, J. D., Norris, A. H., and Shock, N. W. (1976). The effect of age on creatinine clearance in man: a cross-sectional and longitudinal study. *Gerontology* **31**, 155–63.

Seidl, L. G., Thornton, G. F., Smith, J. W., and Cluff, L. E. (1966). Studies on the epidemiology of adverse drug reactions III. Reactions in patients on a general medical service. *Bull. Johns Hopkins Hosp.* **119**, 299–315.

Stevenson, I. H., Salen, S. A. M., and Shepherd, A. M. M. (1979). Studies on drug absorption and metabolism in the elderly. In *Drugs and the elderly – perspectives in geriatric clinical pharmacology* (ed. J. Crooks and I. H. Stevenson) pp. 51–63. Macmillan, London.

Turbott, J., Norman, T. R., Burrows, G. D., Maguire, K. P., and Davies, B. M. (1980). Pharmacokinetics of nortriptyline in elderly volunteers. *Comm. Psychopharm.* **4**, 225–31.

Vestel, R. E. (1978). Drug use in the elderly: a review of problems and special considerations. *Drugs* **16**, 358–82.

Woodford-Williams, E., Alvarez, A. S., Webster, D., Landless, B., and Dixon, M. P. (1964). Serum protein patterns in 'normal' and pathological aging. *Gerontologia* **10**, 86–99.

6

Drug compliance in the elderly

PETER CROME

The proportion of the population receiving prescription medication rises with age. In their study of general practice prescribing in the Oxford area, Skegg *et al.* (1977) found that 24.3 per cent of women aged 75 and over received 20 or more prescriptions per year, compared to only 1.2 per cent of those in the age range 15–29 years. The corresponding figures for men were 20.2 per cent and 0.5 per cent respectively. The rise for women receiving five or more prescriptions a year was more modest, from 23.1 to 61.2 per cent for the same two age ranges. The commonest drugs prescribed on at least one occasion during the year, for women and men respectively aged 75 and over, included psychotropic drugs (37.7 and 27.2 per cent), cardiac drugs (34.7 and 33.3 per cent), and antibiotics (27.1 and 30.6 per cent).

The circumstances in which the elderly are taking their medication at home have been investigated by Shaw and Opit (1976). They found that half of a randomly selected group of elderly patients, registered with a single general practice, were taking drugs regularly. Of those receiving medication, 32 per cent of men and 45 per cent of women were taking three or more drugs regularly. Forty-three per cent of patients prescribed drugs for congestive cardiac failure had not had any contact with their general practitioner for six months or more, the longest interval since consultation being six years. Shaw and Opit (1976) also related mental test scores with social environment. Dividing patients into three groups according to their mental test score, they found that almost half of those in the lower two groups who were receiving prescription drugs were living alone.

From these and other studies of drug use in the elderly at home (Kiernan and Isaacs 1981; Wandless *et al.* 1979), it is abundantly clear that the potential for the elderly to encounter difficulties with their medication is great, and this is borne out in clinical practice. Discussion of adverse drug effects, which account for about 15 per cent of admissions to geriatric units (Learoyd 1972; Williamson and Chopin 1980), is outside the scope of this chapter. The second major problem is non-compliance.

NON-COMPLIANCE

A number of studies have shown that non-compliance in the elderly is very common. Kiernan and Isaacs (1981) studied 50 patients at home drawn randomly from a single inner-city practice. Comparing the dose as recommended on the bottle or package with the dose the patient said they took, it was found that

TABLE 6.1. *Dose compliance for 198 preparations taken by 50 patients. (From Kiernan and Isaacs 1981).*

	Taking the recommended dose		Taking less than the recommended dose		Taking more than the recommended dose		Total no. of drugs
	No	(%)	No	(%)	No	(%)	
Prescribed drugs taken regularly	61	(64)	29	(30)	6	(6)	96
Prescribed drugs taken occasionally	22	(53)	18	(42)	2	(5)	42
Non-prescribed drugs taken regularly	4	(67)	2	(33)	0		6
Non-prescribed drugs taken occasionally	42	(77)	11	(20)	1	(3)	54
Total	129	(65)	11	(20)	9	(5)	198

65 per cent of patients were taking their drugs correctly, 30 per cent took less than the recommended dose, whilst the remaining 5 per cent took an excessive amount. Compliance was highest for non-prescribed drugs taken occasionally, and lowest for prescribed drugs taken on an as required basis (Table 6.1).

Methods of measurement

Drug compliance can be measured in different ways, the most frequently used being patient interviews, tablet counts, and plasma drug measurements. Not surprisingly measurement by different methods produces different results. Wandless *et al.* (1979) studied drug compliance in 81 patients at home aged 65 and over, who were taking at least one prescribed medication regularly. Compliance was measured by three methods based on: interview, tablet counts, and the general practitioners' prescription records. The percentage of medicines taken accurately, defined as not deviating by more than 10 per cent from absolute adherence, for the three methods of measuring compliance was 73, 47, and 40 per cent respectively.

Broadly similar results were reported by Crome *et al.* (1980) in their study of 51 female patients awaiting discharge from a geriatric unit, who were made responsible for their own medication. Measuring compliance by daily tablet counts, they found that the overall non-compliance rate was 42.3 per cent. One-third of patients took their medication correctly whilst eight (15.7 per cent) failed to take any tablets at all. Half the patients could be described as very poor drug takers, failing to take less than half of their drugs correctly.

Parkin *et al.* (1976) reported on 134 patients with a mean age of 66.2 years who were taking drugs following discharge from hospital. Altogether half their patients were not taking their medication correctly when seen at home 10 days after discharge.

From these studies it is clear that non-compliance can be described as the rule rather than the exception and a physician is deluding himself if he thinks that the mere issue of prescription is sufficient to ensure that the drug is taken. Unfortunately none of these studies was designed primarily to assess the clinical significance of this non-compliance, although Crome *et al.* (1980) reported that none of their hospital patients suffered adversely. It is also interesting to note that in the study of Parkin *et al.* (1976) the 42 patients who had died or who had been re-admitted to hospital when reviewed six months later, did not differ from the remaining patients in respect of either of the degree of non-comprehension about their drug dosage or the degree of non-compliance.

The results of six studies in which factors influencing drug compliance were studied are summarized in Table 6.2. It is not surprising that some inconsistencies were found, because the population studied and the methods of measuring compliance were all different. However, there is general agreement that certain social factors, such as social class, education, marital status, and living alone or with others, which might be thought to be associated with non-compliance, are not, in fact, so associated.

TABLE 6.2. *Factors associated with non-compliance reported in six studies.*

Study	Country	Patients studied	Factors associated with non-compliance	Factors not associated with non-compliance
Bloch *et al.* (1977)	USA	Out-patients with glaucoma	Male. No other medical conditions. Side-effects of treatment. Not associating blindness with glaucoma	Age. Marital status. Education. Living alone or with others. Duration of illness. Desire for additional information about glaucoma or efforts to obtain information
Geersten *et al.* (1973)	USA	Out-patients with arthritis	Waiting too long to see the doctor. Being irritated at waiting to see the doctor. Personal relationship.* Being seen within 30 min*	Length of consultation. Good or bad doctor-patient communication. Pain or discomfort of treatment
Hulka *et al.* (1976)	USA	Out-patients with diabetes and heart failure	Number of drugs. Number of doses/day. Doctor-patient communication	Age. Sex. Education. Marital status. Current activity. Number of people in household. Social class. Duration of disease. Number of concurrent diseases
Kiernan and Isaacs (1981)	England	Elderly subjects at home	Prescribed vs non-prescribed drugs. Complexity of dosage regimens	
Parkin *et al.* (1976)	Scotland	Ex-hospital patients	Number of drugs	Age. Sex. Social isolation. Social class. Education. Understanding of illness and treatment. Difficulties or unpleasantness of treatment. Class of drug. Number of daily doses
Wandless *et al.* (1979)	England	Elderly subjects	Women. Medicine taken several times a day	Age. Mental test score. Social class. Marital status. Living alone. Assistance with tablet taking. Duration since last contact with doctor. Use of memory aids

*Associated with compliance.

Influence of age

In none of the studies summarized in Table 6.2 was age reported to be a factor associated with non-compliance. Since old age is associated with a different spectrum of disease with differing prognoses, direct comparisons with younger patients are difficult. However, even in relatively uncommon conditions such as hypertension in chronic haemodialysis patients, age appears not to be a factor in compliance (Briggs *et al.* 1975). Nemitz (1979) found that patients aged over 80 years did not take digoxin as regularly as younger patients. However, in two other studies age was not related to digoxin compliance (Gundert-Remy *et al.* 1976; Weintraub *et al.* 1973).

Multiplicity of medications

The majority of studies have shown that drug compliance becomes less when the number of drugs the patient is taking increases and the dosage regimen becomes more complex. Thus Kiernan and Isaacs (1981) found that only 6 per cent of drugs prescribed in a dosage of one tablet daily were not taken correctly, compared to 75 per cent when the dosage was one tablet three times daily.

The relationship between compliance and dosage frequency has been studied in more detail by Taggart *et al.* (1981). They randomly allocated patients receiving digoxin 0.25 mg daily, to one of three groups who received the drug either once, twice, or four times daily according to the latin-square design. Although patients taking the drug four times daily complied less well, this difference was small and of doubtful clinical relevance (Table 6.3).

TABLE 6.3. *Digoxin compliance in patients receiving 0.25 mg digoxin daily as one, two, or four doses for two month each. (From Taggart et al. 1981).*

	Dosage frequency (tablets/day)		
	1	2	4
Compliance index*	98.5	96.4	92.2[†]
SEM	1.0	1.6	1.9
Plasma digoxin concentration (nmol/l)	1.32	1.28	1.23
SEM	0.06	0.06	0.08

*Compliance index = $\dfrac{\text{number of tablets taken}}{\text{number of tablets prescribed}} \times 100$.

[†]$p < 0.01$ compared to once and twice daily dosage.

Cost of drugs

In the United Kingdom old-age pensioners do not have to pay for prescription medicines and it has been suggested that if drugs were not free then they would be taken more regularly. In the study of Kiernan and Isaacs (1981) it was found that compliance for non-prescribed medication which has to be bought, was higher than that for free prescribed drugs (77 vs 60 per cent, $p < 0.05$). It is likely, however, that the prescribed and non-prescribed medications belonged to different classes of drug. Direct comparison of free and bought drugs belonging to the same class has been investigated (Hemminki and Heikkilä 1975). These authors found that deviation from the recommended dose was higher when the drug had to be bought, by a factor of three for digitalis, four for diuretics and 2.5 for antihypertensive drugs.

Class of drug

Compliance seems to be higher for more potent drugs. Thus Parkin *et al.* (1976) found that non-compliance was lowest for digoxin, anticoagulants, and steroids and highest for psychotropic drugs and mineral replacements. Hemminiki and Heikkilä (1975) found that what they describe as 'drugs proper' were taken more regularly than drugs prescribed for symptomatic relief. Whether these differences are due to added care over prescribing for serious conditions or to some patient-related factor is not known (see Table 6.4).

TABLE 6.4.   *Compliance with prescription drugs according to class in 217 residents of old-peoples homes. (After Hemminki and Heikkila 1975).*

	Percentage compliance			
	No deviation	Used too little	Used too much	No information
Drugs proper				
Thyroid drugs	100	–	–	–
Antibiotics	95	5	–	–
Digitalis	90	9	1	–
Antidiabetics	84	16	–	–
Diuretics	83	15	1	1
Antihypertensives	75	23	2	–
Symptomatic drugs				
Antihistamines	75	25	–	–
Spasmolytics	55	39	6	–
Vasodilators	50	50	–	–
Plain psychotropics	45	49	3	3
Analgesics	21	79	–	–
All drugs	69	28	2	1

Doctor-patient relationships

The quality of doctor-patient relationships as a determinant of drug compliance appears not to have been studied in the elderly. Indeed it would be difficult to do so since many elderly patients receive their medication without any direct contact with their general practitioner. In one study in which doctor-patient relationships were studied it was found that a good relationship was associated with improved drug compliance in patients with cardiac failure (mean age 63 years), but not in patients with diabetes (mean age 53 years). Geersten *et al.* (1973) studied compliance in patients suffering from chronic arthritis. Although the mean age of their patients was only 52 years, their findings may be of relevance since diseases of old age tend to be long lasting. Surprisingly communication measured by both doctor and patient did not appear to influence compliance, nor did patient evaluation of the quality of treatment received!

IMPROVING COMPLIANCE

Counselling, memory-aids and alternative ways of packaging drugs have all been investigated as potential methods of improving drug compliance in the elderly.

Counselling

Macdonald *et al.* (1977) studied the influence of counselling in 165 patients in a geriatric unit. Before discharge from hospital patients were seen by a clinical pharmacist and taught the name and purpose of the drugs and the dose and time of administration. They were also told to destroy all old medication and not to take other people's drugs. Drug compliance was assessed 1, 6, and 12 weeks after discharge. It was found that compliance in the counselled patients was higher than in a control group of non-counselled patients (Table 6.5). This improvement in compliance was also found in patients with mental test scores below that normally associated with an ability to live independently at home. These authors concluded that a designated member of the staff, preferably a pharmacist, should talk to each patient about their medication prior to discharge from hospital.

TABLE 6.5. *Effect of counselling on drug compliance in 165 patients 12 weeks after discharge from hospital. (From Madconald* et al. *1977).*

Group	Percentage of patients taking medication correctly	
	Mental test score 12 or more	Mental test score less than 12
Counselled	81.0	38.5
Counselled plus memory aids	60.0	24
Uncounselled	34.6	14.7

Counselled vs uncounselled MTS 12 or more, $p < 0.01$; MSQ less than 12, $p < 0.05$.
Counselled plus aids vs uncounselled MTS 12 or more and less than 12, both NS.
Counselled plus aids vs counselled MTS 12 or more and less than 12, both NS.

However, no beneficial effect from counselling was observed in a study of elderly patients attending a geriatric day hospital (Wandless and Whitmore 1981). Unfortunately in this latter study, the counselled group were making fewer errors beforehand in their medication than patients in the control group and this may have influenced the result.

Memory aids

Wandless and Davie (1977) compared the effects of two types of memory aid in patients transferred to a geriatric rehabilitation unit. All were orientated in time and space, had suitable visual acuity and were taking medication regularly. Patients on warfarin, insulin, or other parenteral drugs, those who could not read labels and those scoring less than 12 out of 17 on a mental test score, were excluded from the study. It was found that patients given either a written tear-off calendar or a tablet identity card, made fewer mistakes than a control group given verbal information only (Table 6.6). A calendar chart in which the patient ticks off medication as it is taken, has been found helpful in elderly hypertensives (Gabriel *et al.* 1977). Macdonald *et al.* (1977) found that a tear-off calendar

TABLE 6.6. *Percentage drug errors over 14 days in 46 patients receiving different types of instruction. (From Wandless and Davie 1977)*

Type of instruction	Number of patients	Percentage errors	Percentage sum of two-day errors
Verbal only	15	23.2	28.2
Verbal plus tear-off calendar	17	13.4*	17.9†
Verbal plus card identifying tablets and detailing drug regimen	14	18.0†	21.0†

Reduction in errors compared to verbal instruction group: $*p < 0.005$; $†p < 0.0005$.

improved compliance modestly in counselled patients, but that a card detailing the regimen did not improve compliance further.

Oral contraceptives have been packaged in calendar packs for several years and now other drugs are being presented similarly. This method has one major disadvantage in that a separate pack is required for each drug. Recently a new personal medication programme has been developed in which all the patient's medication for a single week can be assembled into a single calendar pack. The completed pack can be labelled for the days of the week and the time of drug administration. The pack is relatively large, 26.5 by 17.5 cm, and thus is only suitable for patients at home. Although this package may be safer in that it reduces the risk of accidental poisoning, a pilot study in elderly patients failed to show any improvement in compliance, compared with drugs administered in conventional bottles (Crome *et al.* 1982).

Purpose-built boxes

The type of package studied by Crome *et al.* (1982) is not yet available commercially but various types of boxes are. One such, the Dosett, contains 28 separate compartments which allows seven days of drugs to be taken at four separate times during the day. Each dose can be taken out of the box by means of a slide. Although this type of box may improve compliance in the individual patient, in at least one study of elderly hospital in-patients it was not found to be helpful (Crome *et al.* 1980). Packing drugs in special boxes, with or without memory-aid stickers, was not found to improve compliance in a study assessing the effects of pentoxifylline (Spriet *et al.* 1980). These types of aid depend on someone transferring tablets from their original bottles. It is possible, however, that this role could be played by the pharmacist who dispenses the drug. Pharmacists might be more inclined to dispense drugs in memory-aid packages if this were to attract a suitable extra fee.

MAXIMUM COMPLIANCE

The problem of non-compliance to prescribed medication can only arise if the physician decides to issue a prescription. The doctor has a duty to prescribe in a way that will minimize the risk of non-compliance. A suggested set of rules to follow is summarized in Table 6.7.

TABLE 6.7. *Prescribing for maximum compliance*

1. Accurate diagnosis
2. Consider whether drug treatment is indicated
3. Decide beforehand how, and by whom response will be measured
4. Prescribe the minimum number of drugs
5. Simple drug regimen
6. Explain purpose of drug to patient
7. Give written instructions
8. Typed labels on bottles

The importance of accurate diagnosis can not be stressed too highly. Simple investigations should not be withheld from the patient simply because of her age. Thus it should not be assumed that all cases of leg oedema are due to cardiac failure. Having reached as accurate a diagnosis as possible the next step is to consider whether drug treatment is appropriate. In the example already mentioned, that of leg oedema, elevation of the legs whilst resting, and supporting stockings whilst walking, may be just as effective as diuretic drugs. If treatment is to be prolonged than it is important to consider from the outset how response is to be measured. This could be undertaken by the physician, a relative, the community nurse, or the patient herself. If the drug does not work, or is no longer needed it should be stopped. These steps may seem obvious but there are still far too many elderly patients taking medication quite unnecessarily.

Although a simple once-daily dosage regimen is to be preferred this is not always the case. For example, the risk of prolonged hypoglycaemia from the once-daily hypoglycaemic agent chlorpropamide, may be greater than the risk of non-compliance with the thrice-daily alternative drug tolbutamide.

Non-comprehension about drug treatment is common in patients leaving hospital (Parkin *et al.* 1976) and it is desirable that all patients should possess certain minimum information about their drugs (*Drugs and Therapeutic Bulletin* 1981). Some patients will require more detailed information and for this group package inserts may be helpful (Hermann *et al.* 1978). In the elderly, however, there is the risk that giving too much information to the patient may just lead to increasing confusion about the drugs. Information can be given by physicians, pharmacists, nurses, or other health-care workers. Who gives it is not important so long as the advice is accurate and consistent.

Although this chapter has concerned itself with the problems of the elderly there is little evidence that compliance in younger patients is any better. The need to prescribe rationally in order to maximize compliance and minimize side-effects applies to patients of all ages.

REFERENCES

Bloch, S., Rosenthal, A. R., Friedman, L., and Coldarolla, P. (1977). Patient compliance in glaucoma. *Br. J. Ophthal.* **61**, 531–4.
Briggs, W. A., Lowenthal, D. T., Cirksena, W. J., Price, W. E., Gibson, T. P., and Flamenbaum, W. (1975). Propranolol in hypertensive dialysis patients: efficacy and compliance. *Clin. Pharmac. Ther.* **18**, 606–12.

Crome, P., Akehurst, M., and Keet, J. (1980). Drug compliance in elderly hospital patients. Trial of the Dosett box. *Practitioner* **224**, 782–5.
— Curl, B., Boswell, M., Lewis, R. R., and Corless, D. (1982). Assessment of a new type of calendar pack – the 'C-Pak'. Submitted for publication.
Drug and Therapeutic Bulletin (1981). What should we tell patients about their medicines? *Drug Ther. Bull.* **19**, 73–4.
Gabriel, M., Gagnon, J.P., and Bryan, C.K. (1977). Improved patient compliance through use of a daily drug reminder chart. *Am. J. public Hlth* **67**, 968–9.
Geersten, H. R., Gray, R. M., and Ward, J. R. (1973). Patient non-compliance within the context of seeking medical care for arthritis. *J. chronic Dis.* **26**, 689–98.
Gundert-Remy, U., Remy, C., and Weber, E. (1976). Serum digoxin levels in patients of a general practice in Germany. *Eur. J. clin. Pharmac.* **10**, 97–100.
Hemminki, E. and Heikkilä, J. (1975). Elderly people's compliance with prescriptions, and quality of medication. *Scand. J. social Med.* **3**, 87–92.
Hermann, F., Herxheimer, A., and Lionel, N. D. W. (1978). Package inserts for prescribed medicines: what minimum information do patients need? *Br. med. J.* ii, 1132–5.
Hulka, B. S., Cassel, J. C., Kupper, L. L., and Burdette, J. A. (1976). Communication, compliance, and concordance between physicians and patients with prescribed medication. *Am. J. public Hlth* **66**, 847–53.
Kiernan, P. J. and Isaacs, J. B. (1981). Use of drugs by the elderly. *J. R. Soc. Med.* **74**, 196–200.
Learoyd, B. M. (1972). Psychotropic drugs and the elderly patient. *Med. J. Aust.* **1**, 1131–3.
Macdonald, E. T., Macdonald, J. B., and Phoenix, M. (1977). Improving drug compliance after hospital discharge. *Br. med. J.* ii, 618–21.
Nemitz, I. (1979). La prescription de digoxine à la sortie de l'hôpital. Etude de la compliance, *Revue méd. Suisse Romande* **99**, 461–8.
Parkin, D. M., Henney, C. R., Quirk, J., and Crooks, J. (1976). Deviation from prescribed drug treatment after discharge from hospital. *Br. med. J.* ii, 686–8.
Shaw, S. M. and Opit, L. J. (1976). Need for supervision in the elderly receiving long-term prescribed medication. *Br. med. J.* i, 505–7.
Skegg, D. C. G., Doll, R., and Perry, J. (1977). Use of medicines in general practice. *Br. med. J.* i, 1561–3.
Spriet, A., Beiler, D., Dechorgnat, J., and Simon, P. (1980). Adherence of elderly patients to treatment with pentoxifylline. *Clin. Pharmac. Ther.* **27**, 1–8.
Taggart, A. J., Johnston, G. D., and McDevitt, D. G. (1981). Does the frequency of daily dosage influence compliance with digoxin therapy? *Br. J. clin. Pharmac.* **11**, 31–4.
Wandless, I. and Davie, J. W. (1977). Can drug compliance in the elderly be improved? *Br. med. J.* i, 359–61.
— Mucklow, J. C., Smith, A., and Prudham, D. (1979). Compliance with prescribed medicines: a study of elderly patients in the community. *J. R. Coll. gen. Practitioners* **29**, 391–6.
— and Whitmore, J. (1981). The effect of counselling by a pharmacist on drug compliance in elderly patients. *J. clin. hosp. Pharm.* **6**, 51–6.
Weinbtraub, M., Au, W.Y., and Lasagna, L. (1973). Compliance as a determinant of serum digoxin concentration. *J. Am. med. Ass.* **224**, 481–5.
Williamson, J. and Chopin, J. M. (1980). Adverse reactions to prescribed drugs in the elderly: a multi-centre investigation. *Age Ageing* **9**, 73–80.

PART II

Cognitive disorders

7

A peptide for the aged? Basic and clinical studies

R. M. PIGACHE

INTRODUCTION

The synthetic peptide Org 2766 has effects in Man on mood, vigilance, and behaviour. Results from various studies in young and elderly subjects, and in geriatric patients, suggest that this peptide might have clinical applications. Before presenting the evidence for these statements, however, it could be useful to set Org 2766 in a broader context. The pioneering work of De Wied and that of subsequent workers, reviewed by Rigter (see next chapter), shows that the peptide produces a variety of behavioural effects in the rat. A recent review by Van Nispen and Greven (1982) on structure–activity relationships, shows that certain of these effects differ from, while some are shared by, other synthetic and endogenous peptides related to adrenocorticotropin (ACTH) and melano-tropin (MSH). It is, however, widely accepted that the relationship between Org 2766 and endogenous ACTH and MSH peptides explains a substantial part of the activity of Org 2766, i.e. this family of peptides acts upon a common set of neural substrates (even though individual members may have additional properties). It is conceivable, of course, that synthetic sequences like ACTH/-α-MSH$_{4-10}$ and Org 2766 might have modes of action totally unrelated to any properties of ACTH or MSH, but here we shall dwell upon the more likely hypo-thesis that such a connection exists.

CHEMICAL NATURE OF ORG 2766

In Fig. 7.1 the structure of Org 2766 is compared with the natural amino acid sequence of ACTH/α-MSH$_{4-9}$. The evident structural modifications were intro-duced (Greven and De Wied 1973, 1977, 1980; De Wied et al. 1975; Witter et al. 1975) to enhance certain actions and to reduce others (Table 7.1). The profile of activity for Org 2766 in Table 7.1 shows that it is very like ACTH/α-MSH$_{4-10}$ (i.e. ACTH/α-MSH$_{4-9}$ lengthened by a glycine residue at position 10), except for potency differences and an important gain in oral activity, the latter resulting from reduced susceptibility to enzymic attack. However, there is as yet no evidence (Krieger and Martin 1981) that a peptide sequence corresponding to ACTH/α-MSH$_{4-10}$, or to similar very short sequences incorporating ACTH$_{4-7}$ in their core (Greven and De Wied 1973), occurs freely in the pituitary or brain. The demonstration of such fragments in free and active forms, with the proteolytic mechanisms for their production, would be very stimulating. Some encouragement

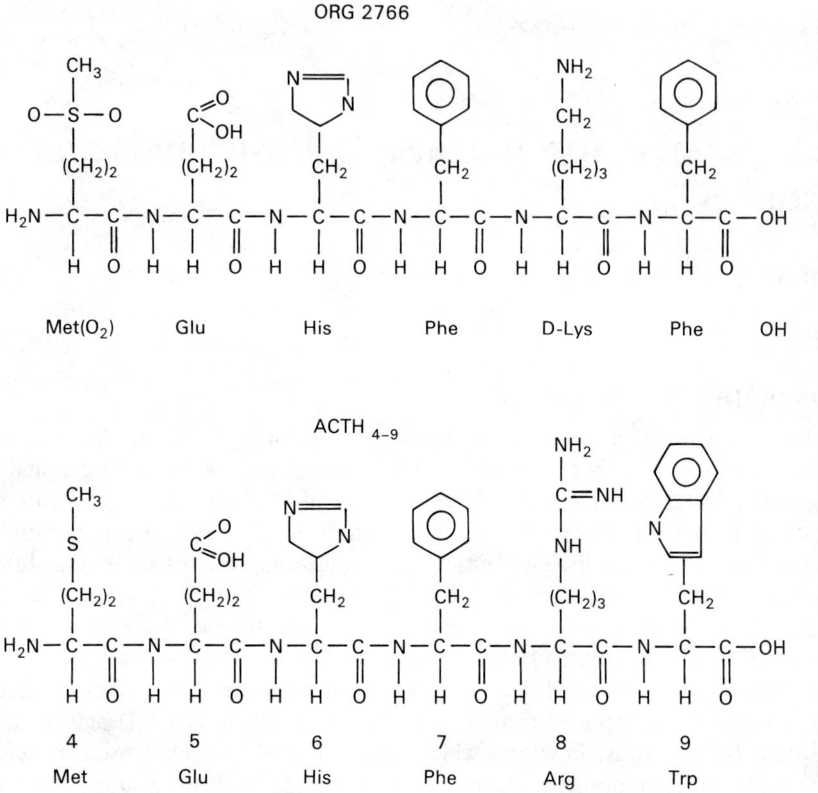

ORG 2766

Met(O$_2$)   Glu   His   Phe   D-Lys   Phe   OH

ACTH $_{4-9}$

4	5	6	7	8	9
Met	Glu	His	Phe	Arg	Trp

Fig. 7.1. Comparison of Org 2766 with the natural sequence of ACTH/α-MSH$_{4-9}$

TABLE 7.1

	ACTH$_{1-24}$	α-MSH$_{1-13}$	ACTH/α-MSH$_{4-10}$	Org 2766
Oral activity	No	No	No	Yes
Resistance to extinction (molar ratio)	1*	Yes	1	× 1000
Enhanced passive avoidance (molar ratio)	Yes	Yes	1*	× 1000
Corticosterone release (activity ratio)				
1. *in vitro*	1*		× 10^{-4}	× 10^{-6}
2. *in vivo*	1*			≃ 0
Melanophore stimulation (activity ratio) *in vivo*	× 10^{-2}	1*	× 10^{-4}	× 10^{-7}
Lypolytic activity	Yes	Yes	Weak	No
Affinity for opiate binding sites (IC$_{50}$ DHM)	× 10^{-6}	Nil	× 10^{-5}	Nil

*Standard.

in this direction stems from the report by Peng Loh and Gainer (1977) of a new, unidentified, small peptide ($\geqslant 700$ Daltons) extracted from both rat pituitary and brain, which possessed potent melanotropic activity. It was speculated that this peptide might have been derived by natural enzymic cleavage from α-MSH. It remains a possibility, of course, that it was a product of the extraction procedure. For the time being, however, it must be assumed that the $ACTH_{4-10}$ sequence normally exerts its influence within the longer amino-acid sequences of naturally-occurring peptides, as it might for example in relation to the lypolytic actions of β-lipotropin (β-LPH) (Schwandt 1981).

Pro-opiomelanocortin derivatives

Recent research by Mains *et al.* (1977), Roberts and Herbert (1977), and Hope and Lowry (1981) has shown that a number of neuropeptides and hormones, already suspected as being related, do indeed stem from a common pituitary prohormone precursor: pro-opiomelanocortin (Pro-OMC). A specification of the amino-acid sequence of this precursor was accomplished by Nakanishi *et al.* (1979). However, the extent to which Pro-OMC is processed, i.e. the fragments it yields, appears to depend essentially on the tissue in which the processing occurs (Krieger and Martin 1981; Watson and Akil 1981*a*).

A schema depicting the differential processing of Pro-OMC within the corticotroph cells of the anterior lobe of the pituitary, and in cells (all) of the intermediate lobe (in species where the intermediate lobe exists), is given in Fig. 7.2. A 'peptide block' representing the $ACTH/\alpha$-MSH_{4-10} sequence is repeated along the bottom of Fig. 7.2 to demonstrate where it recurs in five pituitary Pro-OMC derivatives: $ACTH_{1-39}$, β- and γ-LPH, and α- and β-MSH.

The corticotroph cells of the adenohypophysis process Pro-OMC to $ACTH_{1-39}$ and to β-LPH_{1-93} (Watson and Akil 1980). This pituitary $ACTH_{1-39}$ represents a thousand times more $ACTH_{1-39}$ than is found in the brain (Brownstein 1980; Krieger and Martin 1981). $ACTH_{1-39}$ and β-LPH_{1-93} are both stored together in the same vesicles (Pelletier *et al.* 1977; Weber *et al.* 1979) and are released together by the same hypothalamic factors (for references see Hope and Lowry 1981) into the cavernous sinus and thence into the systemic circulation.

In the intermediate lobe of the pituitary, Pro-OMC is processed further and consequently $ACTH_{1-39}$ becomes a step in the biosynthesis of both α-MSH_{1-13} and 'corticotropin-like intermediate-lobe peptide' ($CLIP_{18-39}$), while β-LPH_{1-93} becomes a step to both γ-LPH_{1-58} and β-endorphin (β-End) (Watson and Akil 1980; Aronin and Krieger 1981). In Man an intermediate lobe as such does not exist, but is represented instead by 'invading cells' scattered in adjacent regions of the anterior and posterior lobes (Celio *et al.* 1980). It has been reported that further processing of $ACTH_{1-39}$ (to α-MSH and CLIP) in human pituitaries occurs solely in fetal and maternal pituitaries (Lowry *et al.* 1977; Visser and Swaab 1977; Aronin and Krieger 1981; Celio *et al.* 1980). However, Kleber *et al.* (1980) have recently isolated immunoreactive α-MSH-like material, which co-eluted with synthetic α-MSH, from both the entire human pituitary and pituitary stalk. It appears that β-LPH_{1-93} is further processed, too, since one of its derivatives (β-End) has been isolated from human pituitaries (Chrétien *et al.*

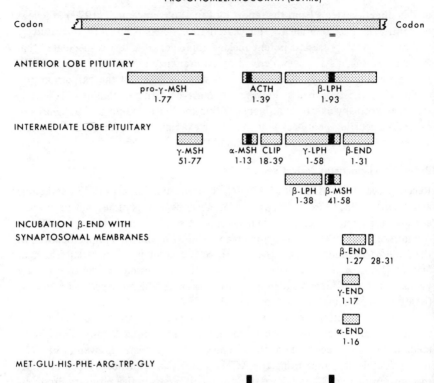

Fig. 7.2. Each short block at the bottom of the figure represents an ACTH/α-MSH$_{4-10}$ sequence and corresponds to locations (shaded black) in fragments of Pro-OMC, shown above, and to sites within Pro-OMC indicated by $=$. Partial representations of the same sequence recurring within Pro-OMC are indicated by $-$. (References in the text except for derivatives obtained from synaptosomal preparations (Burbach *et al.* 1980).)

1977; Li *et al.* 1977) and another (γ-LPH$_{1-58}$) is present in human plasma (Aronin and Krieger 1981). Virtually nothing is known about γ-LPH$_{1-58}$ except that it is the substrate for further cleavage to β-MSH (Chrétien *et al.* 1977; Watson and Akil 1980). Hope and Lowry (1981) have identified β-MSH in sheep intermediate lobe and McLoughlin *et al.* (1980) have identified it in human plasma, but Besser (1981) lately concluded that β-MSH cannot be demonstrated in the human pituitary.

This survey indicates that of the five Pro-OMC derivatives incorporating the ACTH/α-MSH$_{4-10}$ sequence, four are found in the human pituitary. Although the peripheral properties of these hormones (Table 7.2) do not correspond to any known effects of Org 2766, their possible central effects, if known, could suggest mechanisms susceptible to Org 2766. Hence it would be interesting to know if the brain is flooded with pituitary ACTH$_{1-39}$ during stress and at the peaks of circadian output. Central mechanisms responding to these increases might then be triggered by exogenous peptide (Org 2766) administration, here representing a non-physiological augmentation.

TABLE 7.2. *Properties of pituitary hormones incorporating the ACTH/α-MSH$_{4-10}$ sequence*

ACTH	Adrenotropic, melanotropic, lypolytic, glycogenesis, protein synthesis.
α-MSH	Sexual receptiveness, sebaceous gland activity, parturition (Thody 1977) and adrenotropic in the fetus (Challin and Tarosis 1977)
β-MSH	Synthetic peptide strongly melanotropic (Beloff-Chain *et al.* 1977)
β-LPH	Melanotropic, lypolytic, morphinomimetic (Hope and Lowry 1981)
γ-LPH	Unknown

PITUITARY HORMONES IN THE BRAIN

In order to take the above analogy between synthetic and natural Pro-OMC derivatives further, it becomes necessary to ask if pituitary Pro-OMC derivatives can enter the brain to act centrally as neurohormones. Systemically administered ACTH$_{1-39}$, for example, might not cross the blood–brain barrier (Allen *et al.* 1974; Jordan *et al.* 1976) and this is likely to hold for other large peptides.

Much effort in recent years has been put into demonstrating that a route exists to carry substances from the adenohypophysis to the brain. This work has been critically reviewed by Palkovits and Mezey (1981), Mezey *et al.* (1979), and Bergland and Page (1978, 1979). The crux of the matter has been to establish retrograde transport up the long portal vessels to the capillary bed of the median eminence, from whence transport is easier to envisage. The evidence is as follows. First, the necessary vascular connections appear to exist (*op. cit.*). Second, samples of rat portal blood have been shown to contain ACTH, TSH, LH, and PRL which were all abolished by hypophysectomy (Oliver *et al.* 1977). Lastly, radioactivity after [^{3}H]-Org 2766 injection into the pituitary, was found in many brain regions, but primarily in the hypothalamus (Mezey *et al.* 1978). However, the distribution pattern differed from that following intracerebro-ventricular injection (Verhoef *et al.* 1977*a*). In the pituitary study, however, the injection method is likely to have distorted the normal blood-flow pattern (Palkovits and Mezey 1981; Bergland and Page 1978). Retrograde flow under physiological conditions remains difficult to verify.

Once in the capillary bed of the median eminence, pituitary substances could gain access to the brain by various routes. They could leak out locally, e.g. into the arcuate nucleus via fenestrations in the vessel walls (Knigge *et al.* 1973; Rappoport 1976). Also, they could be taken up by tanycytes (making contact with capillary loops), which by reversing their usual direction of transfer would take substances into the cerebrospinal fluid (CSF) of the third ventricle (Bergland and Page 1978; Palkovits and Mezey 1981). Finally, retrograde axonal transport after uptake into local nerve terminals is also a possibility (*op. cit.*).

The circumstantial evidence for retrograde transport of pituitary substances via the portal vessels and their subsequent uptake into brain from the median eminence is inconclusive. It is accepted by many authors and considered by them to be very important, but others are more guarded (Krieger and Liotta 1979). It should be noted, however, that hypophysectomy in the rat results in behavioural deficits. These deficits are not simply explained by a loss of target-organ stimulation, since many can be reversed by a replacement of the pituitary hormones with peripherally-inactive analogues, e.g. ACTH/α-MSH$_{4-10}$ or desglycinamide arginine vasopressin (Bohus and De Wied 1980).

If pituitary Pro-OMC derivatives containing the ACTH/α-MSH$_{4-10}$ sequence enter the CSF as neurohormones, they would diffuse within and around the entire brain. While it is possible that receptors might be similarly widespread, and for Org 2766 to act at all of them, the uptake of Org 2766 after intracerebroventricular (ICV) administration was not diffuse (p. 74), which suggests that this might also be true for the natural Pro-OMC derivatives, i.e. their uptake might be confined to the projection field of Pro-OMC neurons, below.

Pro-OMC in the brain

Pro-OMC derivatives do not disappear from the brain after hypophysectomy (Krieger *et al.* 1977*a, b*; Vaudry *et al.* 1978). This indicates that the brain manufactures the peptides in question on its own account, which probably explains the apparent absence of gross neurological or psychological sequelae following hypophysectomy in Man. There is now, in fact, direct evidence from immunohistochemical methods that neurons within the brain produce β-LPH. The perikarya of these neurons are restricted to scattered cells in the arcuate nucleus, in the ventral border of the hypothalamus and in the supraoptic nucleus (Watson *et al.* 1977). Moreover, these same areas contain cells with ACTH-like immunoreactivity (IR) (Watson *et al.* 1978; Larsson 1977). It was shown later, by sequential-staining methods, that both β-LPH and ACTH-like IR occur in the same cells of the arcuate nucleus and, indeed, within the same vesicles (see references in Watson and Akil 1980). However, Watson and Akil (1981*a*) have reinterpreted this earlier work (including their own) on the basis that cross-reactivity had occurred between ACTH, α-MSH, and CLIP with the antisera used, a criticism voiced earlier by Lowry and Rees (1978). As a result it is now believed that the rat processes β-LPH in the brain as it does in the intermediate lobe of the pituitary (Krieger and Martin 1981; Watson and Akil 1981*a*), producing α-MSH$_{1-13}$, CLIP, γ-LPH$_{1-58}$ and β-End (Fig. 7.2). Also there appears to be a second group of immunoreactive perikarya just lateral to the arcuate nucleus (Akil and Watson 1980; Brownstein 1980; Larsson 1977) which might contain α-MSH not derived from β-LPH$_{1-93}$ ('α-2' MSH neurons). On the other hand, neurons producing solely ACTH, i.e. ACTH *not* as a precursor for α-MSH, might be quite rare in the rat (Krieger and Martin 1981; Larsson 1980). In Man, Kleber *et al* (1980) have identified ACTH$_{1-39}$ and α-MSH-like material in a considerable number of the brain regions listed in the next paragraph. Also, Hosobuchi (1982) has shown that ACTH$_{1-39}$ (and β-End) levels are increased in human CSF (but not in blood) following stimulation of the periaqueductal grey.

Axons stemming from the arcuate Pro-OMC (β-LPH, α-MSH, β-End) neurons have a wide distribution (see references in Watson and Akil 1981*a*; Brownstein 1980; Bloom and Hendrickson 1982). They extend (though in two separate bundles) to rostral limbic structures: amygdala and septal nuclei, interstitial nucleus of the stria terminalis, and nucleus accumbens; and to caudal structures:

hypothalamus, paraventricular nuclei of the dorsal thalamus, substantia nigra, periaqueductal grey, the locus coeruleus, reticular formation, and parabrachial and dorsal raphe nuclei. Very few axons are found in hippocampus, neocortex, or cerebellum (Kendall and Orwoll 1980), and they have not been seen in basal ganglia or spinal cord. Further work could change this picture, of course. This distribution of Pro-OMC derivatives, is remarkably similar to the regional uptake pattern following intracerebroventricular administration of [^{3}H]-Org 2766 (see Table 3 in Verhoef *et al.* 1977*a*). Very recent evidence (Watson and Akil 1981*b*) suggests that the α-2-MSH neurons project to the caudate nucleus, neocortex, and hippocampus.

It is not known if γ-LPH$_{1-58}$ is further processed in the brain to β-MSH. Both peptides contain the ACTH/α-MSH$_{4-10}$ sequence (Fig. 7.2). Watson and Akil (1980) note that β-MSH has been poorly studied in brain, nor is it clear whether it is formed readily or has access to specific high-affinity binding sites.

Central receptors

A crucial element indicating how ACTH/α-MSH$_{4-10}$ and Org 2766 might relate to endogenous ACTH and α-MSH activity, would be knowledge of the possible receptors involved. Watson and Akil (1981*a*) have found ACTH$_{1-39}$ binding sites difficult to demonstrate, although they earlier referred to preliminary data suggesting that ACTH does bind with high affinity, but at very few sites and varying with brain locality (Akil and Watson 1980).

Alpha-MSH receptors have still to be demonstrated (Watson and Akil 1980) and γ-LPH$_{1-58}$ receptors have not yet been looked for (Watson and Akil 1981*a*). If indeed two α-MSH systems exist, that using Pro-OMC as a precursor appears to package its α-MSH in the same vesicles as β-End (Watson and Akil 1980). Accordingly, both substances are released together (Akil and Watson 1980). So it may be assumed that their respective binding sites might lie in close proximity and, of course, β-End has high-affinity opiate receptors (*op. cit.*). As discussed by the foregoing authors, the suggested simultaneous release of two neuromodulators at a synapse challenges Dale's principle of one neuron: one transmitter, but Hökfelt *et al.* (1980) have already shown this to be a less tenable proposition. It should be noted, too, that a separate set of receptors might respond to the α-MSH released by those neurons presumed to produce α-MSH only.

It is generally assumed that ACTH and α-MSH binding sites will be identified within the brain (Jacquet 1978; Wiegant *et al.* 1981; Walker *et al.* 1981). Information on the location and possible variety of these receptors is urgently needed. In addition we need to understand the possible inter-relationship between ACTH/α-MSH receptors and those for co-released β-End, and also for other products possibly derived from β-End at synapses (Fig. 7.2) which might even include des-tyr-γ-endorphin (Van Ree and De Wied 1981).

Org 2766 in the brain

The very reliable effects on rat behaviour (see Chapter 8) and the consistent results on human vigilance (Pigache and Rigter 1981) produced by ACTH- and

MSH-related peptides, including orally administered Org 2766, suggest that these peptides enter the brain. Moreover, behavioural effects in rats resulting from subcutaneous ACTH/α-MSH$_{4-10}$ or Org 2766, can be induced by one-hundredth of the doses used, when the peptides are introduced intracerebroventricularly (Greven and De Wied 1980). In addition, antisera to synthetic α-MSH or ACTH$_{1-24}$ administered ICV, produce behavioural effects that are opposite to those obtained when the peptides themselves are given parenterally (Van Wimersma Greidanus *et al.* 1978). Further circumstantial evidence may be adduced from a reduced septal threshold for driving hippocampal theta activity (Valero *et al.* 1977), from an upward shift in mean hippocampal theta frequency (Urban and De Wied 1976) after parenteral ACTH$_{4-10}$, from enhanced glucose utilization after chronic intraperitoneal (i.p.) Org 2766 treatment (p. 78) and from effects on cyclic adenosine monophosphate following Org 2766 i.p. (p. 76). Lastly, chronic (two-week) administration of ACTH/α-MSH$_{4-10}$ s.c. was shown to reduce the number of corticosterone-binding sites in the hippocampus (De Kloet *et al.* 1980).

Many relatively small peptides have been said to enter the brain after peripheral administration, viz. α-MSH (Greenberg *et al.* 1976), MIF-1 (Greenberg *et al.* 1976; Pelletier *et al.* 1975), arginine vasopressin (Greenberg *et al.* 1976), and Org 2766 (Mezey *et al.* 1978). However, these studies measured uptake in terms of total radioactivity only, this being not necessarily the same as intact peptides. For Org 2766 (as intact peptide) whole-brain uptake in the rat after intravenous administration corresponded to an average of 0.01 per cent of the administered dose, found 30 min after administration (Verhoef and Witter 1976). Following oral administration approximately one-hundredth of the latter value was found.

Verhoef, Palkovits and Witter (1977*a*) introduced [^{3}H]-Org 2766 ICV, to map its distribution in the rat brain. Regions where radioactivity due to the intact peptide or its metabolites scored high, comprised arcuate and certain other hypothalamic nuclei, interstitial nucleus of the stria terminalis, periaqueductal grey, locus coeruleus, and the septal nuclei (where levels became very high in the dorsal and fimbrial nuclei). This results in further indirect evidence that Org 2766 might enter the brain, since ACTH/α-MSH$_{4-10}$ and ACTH$_{1-24}$ when administered subcutaneously were able to prevent the septal binding of Org 2766 introduced ICV (Verhoef *et al.* 1977*b*), i.e. because these natural peptide sequences apparently passed from blood to brain, so might Org 2766. The low dose levels of Org 2766 needed to produce behavioural effects and the minute percentages (see above) reaching the brain suggest that high affinity/low capacity receptors might exist in very small regions of brain.

Before reaching the brain, after oral administration, Org 2766 has to overcome several physiological barriers. The impact of some of these barriers on the stability of Org 2766 has been investigated:

after 6 h *in vitro* incubation of Org 2766 in human gastric juice 90–95 per cent Org 2766 had remained unchanged (Organon, unpublished data);

after 6 h *in vitro* incubation in human intestinal juice approximately 30 per cent Org 2766 was unchanged (*op. cit.*);

after intravenous administration of Org 2766 to rats and dogs, the half-lives of elimination were found to be 16 and 30 min, respectively (*op. cit.*) or in another study (Verhoef and Witter 1976) 4 min in the rat;

oral dosing of Org 2766 to conscious rats gave maximal peak plasma levels between 1-4 h after administration (Verhoef and Witter 1976);

tentatively, the *in-vitro* half-life in human plasma was found to be approximately 60 min (Organon, unpublished data);

after oral dosing it seems probable that Org 2766 has been identified in human plasma (Forsman, report to Organon; Organon, unpublished data).

MECHANISMS OF ACTION OF ORG 2766

Neurotransmitter modulation

The effects of ACTH, MSH, and certain synthetic analogues of these peptides on neurotransmitter metabolism have been the subject of extensive and critical reviews (Dunn and Gispen 1977; Versteeg 1981). A variety of effects have been reported. However, certain similarities between these peptides, in terms of neurotransmitter metabolism, were discounted by Versteeg (1980) as possible direct explanations for the behavioural effects in the rat. This was largely because some synthetic analogues share effects on neurotransmitters and passive avoidance, but have opposite effects to each other on active avoidance. Also, Org 2766 (100 µg/kg daily for two weeks) shares many of the behavioural but none of the transmitter interactions of $ACTH_{1-24}$, i.e. Org 2766 did not affect total brain noradrenalin, dopamine, or serotonin turnover (Organon, unpublished data). Likewise, it did not increase hippocampal acetylcholine turnover, as was seen with $ACTH_{1-24}$ or α-MSH (where it was associated with the 'stretching, yawning syndrome') when all peptides were given ICV (Wood *et al.* 1978). On the other hand, using an unusual and subtle technique, Lichtensteiger and Monnet (1979) showed that Org 2766 i.p. decreased the firing rate of nigral dopaminergic neurons, but had only a slight effect on arcuate neurons. Thus many more studies, looking especially at regional variations, are needed before confident conclusions can be reached concerning, behaviourally relevant, neurotransmitter modulation by ACTH-like peptides, including Org 2766.

Interaction with opiate mechanisms

Intracerebroventricular injections of morphine and certain Pro-OMC derivatives including: β-End, $ACTH_{1-24}$, and α-MSH (Wiegant *et al.* 1977*b*), and β-MSH (Gispen *et al.* 1975), induce 'grooming behaviour' in the rat which can be blocked by naloxone, suggesting action at a stereo-specific opiate receptor. On the other hand, it should be noted that *in vitro* $ACTH_{1-24}$ (Table 7.1) has only a slight affinity for dihydromorphine (DHM) receptors and α-MSH none (Wiegant *et al.* 1977*b*). Also, $ACTH_{1-24}$-induced 'grooming' can be blocked by haloperidol (Wiegant *et al.* 1977*a*), suggesting, too, an action at dopamine sites. Org 2766 has no affinity *in vitro* for DHM binding sites (cited in De Wied *et al* 1978; Organon, unpublished data), nor any for leu-enkephalin or etorphin sites (Witter, report to Organon; Organon, unpublished data). Nor does it induce excessive grooming (Gispen *et al.* 1975). A rapid extinction of pole-jump avoidance induced by naltrexone was apparently reversed by Org 2766 (De Wied *et al.* 1978). However, at all dose levels of naltrexone the delay of extinction produced by Org 2766 related to the dose of peptide given, but higher doses of naltrexone did *not* require increased Org 2766 to delay extinction. Accordingly, Org 2766 appears not to have acted as a competitive antagonist for naltrexone binding sites, but rather to have operated via independent mechanisms.

Org 2766 has no effect in traditional tests used for screening analgesic drug effects (Organon, unpublished data). These findings do not conflict with the recent report that at very high, non-physiological, doses, Org 2766 (3-30 μg, injected directly into the periaqueductal grey) induced analgesia (Walker *et al.* 1981). Moreover, the analgesia with Org 2766 was not like that produced by β-End, in that it could not be blocked by naloxone.

Thus Org 2766 seems not to affect opiate mechanisms. The highly complex web of interactions, between ACTH, MSH, and similar peptides and opiate receptors, and between morphine and ACTH receptors (Jacquet 1978) is a separate issue that needs to be resolved.

Second messenger mechanisms

Wiegant *et al.* (1981) have recently reviewed the literature relating to cyclic adenosine monophosphate (cAMP) and to protein phosphorylation, as influenced by ACTH peptides. The following brief account tries to connect this work to Org 2766.

Wiegant *et al.* (1979) present evidence that low concentrations of $ACTH_{1-24}$, *in vitro*, stimulate adenylate cyclase, whereas high doses (10^{-4} M or greater) are inhibitory. At 10^{-4} M (the only dose level tested) $ACTH_{1-10}$ and ACTH/α-MSH_{4-10} had no effect on adenylate cyclase activity. On the other hand, at a lower dose, $ACTH_{1-10}$ (10^{-5} M) produced a 50 per cent increase in basal cAMP levels in rat brain slices containing the N. parafascicularis (Wiegant and Gispen 1975), a structure involved in ACTH/α-MSH behavioural effects (Bohus and De Wied 1967). However, in contrast to the *in vitro* inhibition of adenylate cyclase by high doses of ACTH, high doses (5-50 μg intrathecally) of ACTH, or α-MSH, given *in vivo* increased CSF concentrations of cAMP (Rusman and Isaacs 1975). Chronic treatment with α-MSH also increased cAMP levels in the occipital cortex of rats (Christensen *et al.* 1976). Since a single *in vivo* ('low') dose, higher than that needed to affect avoidance behaviour, of another fragment $ACTH_{1-16}NH_2$ (1 μg ICV), also increased cAMP in the septum, neocortex, cerebellum, and substantia nigra, but reduced it in the basal ganglia, Wiegant *et al.* (1979) stressed the importance of the N-terminal portion of $ACTH_{1-24}$ in stimulating adenylate cyclase. At the same time they noted a small, but similar, contribution from the short ACTH/α-MSH_{4-7} sequence.

Clearly, there appear to be differences in relation to dose effects between *in vitro* and *in vivo* preparations, differences between ACTH fragments and different responses between brain regions. There could be, too, differences between acute and chronic peptide treatments. Furthermore, Daly (1977) has commented on the wide variation in the results of drug studies on the cAMP

TABLE 7.3. *Percentage difference in the cAMP content of various mouse brain areas at times indicated after Org 2766 (40 µg/kg i.p.) compared with control = 100 per cent. (Data calculated from (1) Schneider et al. (1981), (2) Schneider, Felt, and Goldman (Manuscript to Organon 1981), (3) Schneider et al. (1977).)*

Time post Org 2766:	10 min		30 min			1 h		4 h	24 h	
Sex:	M	M	M	M	F	M	M	M	M	F
Reference:	(3)	(2)	(1)	(2)	(1)	(3)	(2)	(2)	(1)	(1)
Brain area:										
Olfactory bulbs	—	+33*	—	+16	- 4	—	-35*	+10	—	-51*
Septum	—	-29*	—	+ 2	+ 9	—	-48*	+10	-18*	-39*
Hippocampus	—	- 4	—	+ 6	+11	+ 80*	-17*	+ 6	+20*	-38*
Hypothalamus	—	- 2	—	-30*	- 8	—	-40*	+ 2	—	-29*
Midbrain	—	-13	+22*	+ 5	0	+130*	-20*	- 6	—	-18
Thalamus	—	+ 6	—	- 2	+12	—	-28*	- 2	+24*	-28*
Frontal cortex	+147	- 1	—	+ 9	+ 9	—	-39*	+24	—	-21
Parietal cortex	—	+16	—	- 1	+18	—	-32*	+14	+27*	-26*
Occipital cortex	—	-13	—	+18	-12	—	-23*	+ 8	—	-43*
Striatum	+181	+16	—	+ 9	+ 8	+141*	- 5	+14	—	-31
Cerebellum	—	+50*	+29	+ 4	- 2	+140*	-27*	- 9	—	-23
Medulla/pons	—	0	—	+ 4	+13	—	-42*	+ 6	·	-42*

— No data given;   *$p < 0.05$ max.

system. Sources of variation as above, or relating otherwise to methods, might account for a lack of consistency in the results of Schneider and his colleagues (Table 7.3). Schneider *et al.* (1981*a*) suggest, too, the possibility of a sexual dimorphism to explain their findings. However, the human behavioural data they cite to support this contention do not inspire confidence (*op. cit.*). It is evident that more data with Org 2766 are needed, especially in relation to chronic dosing. Even then it might be difficult to establish that an observed effect (stimulation or inhibition of adenylate cyclase) was necessarily a direct effect of the peptide. The adenylate cyclase system could be stimulated indirectly, e.g. via neurotransmitters modulated in some other way by the peptides. It will also be necessary to show the behavioural relevance of any such effects.

It was found, too, by Wiegant and colleagues (*op. cit.*) that $ACTH_{1-24}$ and related fragments appear to inhibit membrane-bound protein kinases. The authors therefore propose a new 'second messenger' model to take account of this result, whereby after ACTH/receptor binding or treatment with ACTH/α-MSH fragments there is a modulation of membrane-bound protein kinases, resulting in reduced protein phosphorylation and leading to a presumed change in the conformation of membrane phospholipids, thus allowing calcium (Ca^{2+}) to enter the cell. This Ca^{2+} in its role as a second messenger would then regulate the activity of intracellular enzymes, with many possible physiological consequences. They further suggest that this mechanism might underlie the 'excessive grooming' behaviour produced by certain ACTH fragments. However, in so far as the last proposal is substantiated, the mechanism does not account for Org 2766 effects since this analogue does not induce 'excessive grooming'. It may be hoped that direct information on Org 2766 and protein kinase inhibition will be forthcoming.

Cerebral glucose metabolism

Single doses of Org 2766 given to male mice (10 µg/kg s.c.) had no effect on the uptake of $[^3H]$-2-deoxyglucose given 10 min after the peptide and 45 min prior to decapitation (Delanoy and Dunn 1978). This contrasts with the findings after chronic peptide treatment. McCulloch *et al.* (1981) treated male rats with Org 2766 (100 µg/kg i.p. for 10 days). Glucose utilization was then measured by $[^{14}C]$-2-deoxyglucose uptake and autoradiography. Of 49 discrete brain areas examined, statistically significant increases in uptake after Org 2766, as compared with placebo, were found in four discrete brain regions: anterior nucleus of the thalamus, anterior cingulate cortex, parasubiculum, and the molecular layer of the hippocampus. This distribution does not necessarily indicate the primary site of action for Org 2766, but it represents a coherent neural circuit within the limbic system. The parasubiculum provides major hippocampal projections to the mamillary nuclei and anterior thalamus (Swanson and Cowan 1977). The mamillary nuclei also project to the anterior thalamic nucleus, and the latter nucleus is reciprocally connected with the anterior cingulate gyrus. This limbic circuit is well selected to mediate motivational and/or attentional processes. Work is now needed with those analogues of ACTH/MSH that have other behavioural profiles (e.g. $[D\text{-}Phe_7]$-$ACTH_{4-10}$) to determine the significance of the findings with Org 2766. In addition, it will be interesting to establish the site of actions of the peptide yielding the observed metabolic effects.

Neurotrophic effects

There is a new and growing literature on ACTH-like peptides producing enhanced regeneration in peripheral nerves and preventing age-related degeneration in the central nervous system. These various trophic effects were found after chronic peptide treatments.

$ACTH_{1-24}$ and the non-corticotrophic peptides: $ACTH_{1-10}$, $ACTH/\alpha\text{-}MSH_{4-10}$, and $\beta\text{-}MSH$, all increase the incorporation of amino acids into brain proteins (see reviews by Dunn and Gispen 1977; Gispen *et al.* 1977; Bohus and De Wied 1980). ACTH also modulates the electrophysiological properties of motor neurons (Strand *et al.* 1973/74; Strand *et al.* 1976; Strand *et al.* 1977), and increases the frequency of preterminal branching in motor endplates (Shapiro *et al.* 1968). Accordingly, Strand and Kung (1980) studied the effects of chronic (three-week) $ACTH_{1-39}$ administration (s.c.) upon neuromuscular regeneration in adrenalectomized male rats following crush injury to the sciatic nerve. They found that the hormone promoted axonal growth, increased both the number of large motor endplates and preterminal branching, and resulted in a more rapid functional recovery, i.e. both sensorimotor (footflick to heat stimulation) and motor (walking, holding and toe spread). They suggested that the hormone acts here primarily on motor neurons, probably by both modulating their excitatory state and influencing protein synthesis in the cell bodies for transport along the axons.

Support for the above findings comes from a study by Bijlsma *et al.* (1981). They treated endocrinologically-intact female rats with long-acting preparations of $ACTH_{1-24}$, $ACTH/\alpha\text{-}MSH_{4-10}$ or Org 2766 by subcutaneous injections on alternate days. Significant recovery of the footflick response following sciatic nerve crush occurred sooner and in a dose-related manner under all treatments, as compared to the controls. These authors, too, speculate that the effect might stem from enhanced protein synthesis.

A conceivably related trophic action of ACTH-like peptides is an apparent retardation of certain age-related degenerative changes in the rat hippocampus. In this structure, reactive astrocytes, evidenced by hypertrophied somata and thickened processes, occur as a manifestation of age (Landfield *et al.* 1977; Lindsey *et al.* 1979) and their mean density has been shown to correlate directly with age (Landfield *et al.* 1978*b*). Similar astrocytes are found in human senile (neuritic) plaques (Wisniewski and Terry 1973). In Man, the mean neuron density of the hippocampus was significantly and negatively correlated with 'normal' aging, but in Alzheimer's disease the rate was far more steep (Ball 1977; also Tomlinson and Henderson 1976). This cell loss was exponentially correlated with the number of remaining neurons exhibiting neurofibrillary tangles or granulovacuolar degeneration.

A pituitary–adrenal connection with hippocampal aging has been suggested by Landfield *et al.* (1978*b*), who found that, in the rat, the reactive astrocyte count, and also a total glial/astrocyte count, correlated positively with plasma corticosterone concentrations and with adrenal weight in aged animals. Moreover, Landfield *et al.* (1978*a*) reported that adrenal-weight suppression, used as a

80   *A peptide for the aged? Basic and clinical studies*

bioassay for *effective* glucorticoid activity, produced by chronic administration (7.5 months) of corticosterone, correlated highly with astrocyte hypertrophy. By contrast, adrenalectomy (Landfield *et al.* 1979) retarded brain aging, as indicated by microglia, astrocyte inclusions, and reduced neuronal density. It is therefore extremely interesting that Landfield *et al.* (1981) have now shown that adrenalectomy at 18 months of age significantly increased the neuronal packing density in the hippocampi of rats sacrificed nine months later, as compared to age-matched controls. Furthermore, chronic treatment (s.c.) with either Org 2766 or the neural stimulant pentylenetetrazole (PTZ), for 10 months after the age of 16 months, significantly increased the neuronal packing density and also decreased astrocyte reactivity, as compared with the aged controls. In these respects the aged controls also differed from young control animals. The drugs also improved reversal learning on testing 8.5 months after treatment. Thus Org 2766 and PTZ exerted long-term trophic effects on brain structure and function.

In rat brain by far the highest extent of corticosterone binding occurs in the hippocampus, followed by that in the septum (Knizley 1972; McEwen *et al.* 1972; Stumpf and Sar 1975). This binding is highly specific (McEwen *et al.* 1976; De Kloet *et al.* 1975). Corticosterone binds in the cytosol, and the corticosterone-receptor complex is taken up by the cell nuclei (McEwen *et al.* 1975). The complex acts at the genome making portions of DNA accessible to enzymes and their substrates, thus enabling transcription of RNA which can then direct the formation of new protein (De Vellis and Kukes 1973). Also, and most relevant to this and to cerebral glucose metabolism, cell proliferation and transport processes for glucose, nucleotides, and amino acids are all reduced by cortisol and cortisol also inhibits DNA synthesis during postnatal brain development (De Vellis and Kukes 1973). Many central effects of ACTH-like peptides in the rat are opposite to those of corticosterone (see review by Bohus and De Wied 1980). The effects of Org 2766 just noted might be related to a control (reduction) of corticosterone binding in the hippocampus. Such an effect upon *in vitro* cortico-sterone binding was obtained after $ACTH_{1-24}$, or the non-corticotrophic peptide $ACTH/\alpha\text{-}MSH_{4-10}$, had been administered (s.c.) to hypophysectomized rats for two weeks prior to sacrifice (De Kloet *et al.* 1980). The same might occur in intact animals as a response to ACTH of pituitary and/or neuronal origin, as proposed by De Kloet *et al.* (*op. cit.*). It is possible, too, that α-MSH produced in the pituitary or by arcuate neurons, or by the α-2-MSH neurons, would exert a similar control. This action could be direct or mediated indirectly. A manifestation of such control would appear to be an attenuation of processes that otherwise impair function and shorten cell life (cf. Wexler 1976).

Cerebral haemodynamics

Gann *et al.* (1979) recently concluded that 'all neurons that have been responsive to haemodynamic manipulation have been located in [brain] areas implicated in the control of ACTH'. These areas, however, control more hormones than just ACTH. None the less, it is relevant that investigators should have looked at the converse proposition, i.e. for haemodynamic effects of ACTH, to see if ACTH-like peptides in turn affect, for example, regional cerebral blood-flow.

Studies with α-MSH (Goldman *et al.* 1975) and Org 2766 (Goldman *et al.* 1979) in the rat had suggested that these peptides decrease regional cerebral blood-flow (rCBF). However, one requirement for the method employed was that the indicator used (antipyrine) should diffuse freely from capillaries into the brain. It has been shown, however, that antipyrine has limited diffusibility (Eckman *et al.* 1975; Eklöf *et al.* 1974), with the consequence that rCBF determined with antipyrine is likely to be underestimated. Goldman and Murphy (1981) have repeated their earlier work using the more diffusible and lipid-soluble iodoantipyrine (Sakurada *et al.* 1978). They included again antipyrine, but exploited this time its limited diffusibility to provide a measure of capillary permeability. The previously observed decrease in rCBF no longer obtained and at every location could be explained by a reduced extraction of the antipyrine in the former studies. In the new study Org 2766, given i.v. to male rats, did *not* affect blood-flow significantly in any of the eleven regions examined. However, the uptake of antipyrine was significantly reduced in hypothalamus, hippocampus, and in parietal and frontal cortices. Moreover, Org 2766 has lately been found to reduce the extraction of two more, quite different, diffusion-limited substances: caffeine and morphine (Goldman, personal communication). How such localized decreases in extraction would occur is not understood. The authors suggest a decreased capillary permeability, but this in turn would require an, as yet unspecified, intermediary mechanism since it seems rather improbable that the minute concentrations of Org 2766 in plasma would be sufficient to cover the area of capillary endothelium implicated. It is difficult to judge the real significance of these observations. Further information on the results of chronic peptide treatment could be most interesting.

Summary

It is evident from the foregoing that the mechanisms of action of Org 2766 are not understood, but that many avenues have been opened for further exploration. It is of paramount importance to identify and locate the ligands for Org 2766. Otherwise the most promising leads might be those relating to second messenger systems and to energy metabolism, probably restricted to specific neural circuits, and to mechanisms mediating the neurotrophic actions. Although not mentioned earlier, the possibility of an action not involving a second messenger should be considered. Thus endocytosis of the neurohormone–receptor complex, with subsequent release of the internalized neurohormone, could occur (King and Cuatrecasas 1981), which might apply also to an analogue such as Org 2766. Despite the many questions outstanding, it does seem that we can conclude at this stage that Org 2766 influences neuronal function(s).

ORG 2766 EFFECTS IN MAN

The numerous studies on ACTH/α-MSH$_{4-10}$ (Org 01 63) and Org 2766 in man have been evaluated in several recent reviews (Gaillard 1980; Pigache and Rigter 1981; Pigache 1982). The presentation here tries not to duplicate the available detailed discussions, but concentrates instead on material that was either insufficiently dealt with earlier, or that is new. The original hypotheses for ACTH peptide effects in man represented extrapolations from particular interpretations of the animal data. The idea that these peptides temporarily (i.e. within hours after their administration) increase the motivational value of environmental stimuli, resulting possibly in greater selective attention (Beckwith and Sandman 1978), has been a constant theme (for reviews see: Bohus and De Kloet 1979; De Kloet and De Wied 1980). In addition, the evidence that memory retrieval in the rat might be facilitated, too, would seem to require just a slight adjustment in the theory (Rigter and Crabbe 1979). However, it can be stated quite definitely that so far the above peptides have not had any effect on human memory (Pigache 1982). Possible reasons for this have been discussed (*op. cit.*). Nor have the peptides affected a variety of tests possibly related to perception (*op. cit.*), but this might reflect on the test methods used. Areas where positive effects have been seen are reviewed below.

Arousal

Neither ACTH/α-MSH$_{4-10}$ nor Org 2766 has shown an affect on general arousal, which is consistent with the animal data (Bohus 1981). This has been demonstrated many times in relation to critical flicker fusion (Pigache 1981) and to simple reaction time, tracking, and finger-tapping tasks in a wide variety of healthy volunteers and patients (Hornsveld and Zwaan, report to Organon; Will *et al.* 1978; Branconnier *et al.* 1979; Schneider *et al.* 1981*b*; Ferris and Reisberg 1981). It applies, too, to psychophysiological variables recorded under basal conditions (Pigache and Rigter 1981). The spontaneous EEG analysed by computer methods, also failed to show any effects of the peptides in either healthy young volunteers or elderly subjects, even after chronic dosing (reviewed in Pigache and Rigter 1981). A report (Branconnier *et al.* 1979) of EEG effects (especially relating to alpha) in the elderly after acute ACTH$_{4-10}$ is inconclusive since no main treatment effects were observed. Also, no significant changes were seen in the sleep EEGs of young healthy volunteers after doses of Org 2766 as high as 120 mg, although caffeine citrate (300 mg) had clear-cut effects (Nicholson and Stone 1980).

Increased arousal related to task performance, however, does seem to be fairly consistent with both peptides. This was seen for forearm blood-flow (Breier *et al.* 1979), where the effect also interacted with personality variables, for heart rate (Rockstroh *et al.* 1981; Fehm-Wolfsdorf *et al.* 1981) and heart-rate variability (reviewed in Pigache and Rigter 1981), and for the Achilles tendon reflex (Brunia and Van Boxtel 1978).

Attention

Short-duration tests of attention for the most part have not been successful in showing effects of the ACTH peptides (see review by Pigache and Rigter 1981), but it might be that these tests are relatively insensitive to drugs, especially to non-sedative drugs.

A test of selective attention used in five studies with ACTH peptides required the learning of a simple discrimination to a criterion and then its relearning: first after reversal (R) of the reward contingencies, then after an intradimensional shift (IDS), and finally after an extradimensional shift (EDS). A model of selective attention proposed by Sutherland (1959) and Lovejoy (1966), for infrahuman species, predicts that treatments which enhance selective attention will result in an earlier acquisition of R. An extension of the model, by Zeaman and House (1963), predicts that such treatments will also enhance IDS and impair EDS. In a much-cited study, Sandman *et al.* (1975) reported that healthy male volunteers performed the IDS problem less well *during* an infusion of $ACTH_{4-10}$ than one hour *afterwards*, whereas EDS performance was better during performance than after. There was no significant main effect of treatment, only the *pattern* of changes differed significantly between treatments. Moreover, the required effect for R was not obtained. None the less, the authors interpreted the results as the effect of $ACTH_{4-10}$ causing hypoattention during infusion and hyperattention afterwards. A subsequent, similar, study (Sandman *et al.* 1977) also failed to satisfy any of the above predictions. Healthy females, tested during menstruation or at midcycle, were even significantly *impaired* by $ACTH_{4-10}$ during reversal learning, relative to placebo. This result runs counter to that predicted by the model. There were no significant effects on IDS or EDS. Mentally retarded males tested after infusions of $ACTH_{4-10}$ or placebo provided no significant between-treatment group effects in relation to the model (Sandman *et al.* 1976), nor did retardates treated with Org 2766 (Walker and Sandman 1979). It can be concluded therefore that the above test procedures failed to show any consistent effect of the ACTH peptides. It should be added, perhaps, that in three of the studies (Sandman *et al.* 1976, 1977; Walker and Sandman 1979) further analyses of subproblems within the EDS phase were undertaken. These data, however, relate to another aspect of performance (Tighe *et al.* 1971), i.e. concept learning, but this, too, requires the same changes in R and IDS, as above, which were not observed.

The EEG has been used to assess the effects of ACTH peptides on mechanisms related to attention. According to Endroczi *et al.* (1970) $ACTH_{1-24}$ attenuated EEG alpha activity (desynchronization or alpha-blocking) during an overlearned task, i.e. it caused dishabituation. This was not replicated by Brunia (report to Organon), but was apparent during a vigilance study by O'Hanlon (first report to Organon) where Org 2766, relative to placebo, reduced 8–13 Hz activity while improving vigilance. It was seen, too, with $ACTH_{1-24}$ which caused desynchrony to recur after alpha activity (recorded between the warning and imperative stimuli of a disjunctive reaction time task) had become re-established, i.e. after habituation had ensued (Miller *et al.* 1974). In a task very like the last, however, Rockstroh *et al* (1981) obtained the opposite result, i.e. Org 2766 increased 8–10 Hz and decreased 12–14 Hz activity during the interstimulus interval, as a function of trials. The findings are difficult to reconcile with each other.

EEG average evoked responses (AERs) occur in the interval between a warning stimulus (S1) and an imperative stimulus (S2) requiring a motor response that terminates S2, and include within their complex waveform an early negative component, occurring at about 100 ms after S1 (N 100) and a late positive component at about 300 ms (P 300). The former has been connected with a process subserving the detection/selection of simple cue characteristics (Hillyard *et al.* 1978; Parasuraman and Beatty 1980), and the second with stimulus evaluation/categorization in relation to a neural template (Hillyard *et al.* 1978; Parasuraman and Beatty 1980; McCarthy and Donchin 1981). Two studies based on such a constant foreperiod (6 s) reaction time paradigm used: identical subject inclusion criteria (healthy young volunteers), setting, equipment, methods of data collection and analysis, and similar stimulus (auditory) characteristics and the same response (depression of a single microswitch). The first study (Rockstroh *et al.* 1981), used one pair of S1/S2 stimuli and found, amongst other effects, that Org 2766, compared with placebo, resulted in faster reaction times ($p < 0.05$), shorter N 100 latencies ($p < 0.05$) and a trend towards greater P 300 amplitudes ($p < 0.1$). The second study (Fehm-Wolfsdorf *et al.* 1981) varied the procedure by using two different pairs of S1/S2 stimuli, with the S2 of one pair being an aversively loud sound. The results in relation to Org 2766 were contrary to the first study, i.e. longer reaction times ($p < 0.01$), though less so for the aversive S2 than for the neutral S2, and a decreased P 300 amplitude ($p < 0.05$). The authors interpret their two studies as a facilitation of selective attention (i.e. the processing of relevant stimuli) by Org 2766 in the first study, where a single attentional set had to be maintained, but impairing selection/categorization in the second study where subjects had to switch between two different attentional sets differing in quality and relevance. The reality of this switching is substantiated by the fact that though subjects were required to make one and the same motor response in both studies, their reaction times were longer in the second, even under placebo, and were lengthened less for the aversive S2, indicating that they made contingent responses. The reduced P 300 in the second study was explained on the basis that randomness in the sequence of stimulus pairs, compelled subjects constantly to switch between the two sets and so put a burden on them. This might have caused some stress, as evidenced by a concomitant decrease in heart rate, especially under Org 2766. Thus Org 2766 would seem to have enhanced the fixation of attention at the apparent cost of impairing its switching. The above observations are being repeated in a single group of subjects as a further test of this challenging hypothesis.

Although no results for N 100 in the above successive ('go, go') discrimination task were reported by Fehm-Wolfsdorf *et al* (1981), an earlier study (Miller *et al.* 1976) found that in a visual continuous performance task, involving a successive 'go, no-go' discrimination, $ACTH_{4-10}$ s.c. resulted in significantly longer latencies and decreased amplitudes for an early negative component in the AER (occurring at about 200 ms). A recent evoked potential study by Sandman *et al.* (in press) using simple 20 ms light flashes, failed to find any dose-related, or significant main effects, with either Org 2766 or dexamphetamine treatments. It is evident that the task requirements are an important factor in showing AER effects of the peptides.

Vigilance

A study involving healthy young volunteers (Gaillard and Sanders 1975) and another in hypophysectomized patients (Gaillard and Hornsveld, report to Organon) used $ACTH_{4-10}$. A third study in young volunteers (Gaillard and Varey

1979) used three levels of Org 2766. In all three studies the peptides consistently and significantly prevented the occurrence of a time-on-task decrement in serial reaction time performance (self-paced), as seen with placebo. Such a decrement can be regarded as the build up of reactive inhibition, but more often it is ascribed to lapses of attention possibly related to failing motivation.

O'Hanlon (first report to Organon) gave a lengthy vigilance task, involving a brightness discrimination, to similar volunteers and found that Org 2766 (40 mg) and dexamphetamine (10 mg) equally and significantly prevented a time-related decrement in the percentage of targets hit correctly, which did occur with placebo (Fig. 7.3). He failed, however, to replicate this finding (using Org 2766 only) in elderly, retired volunteers (O'Hanlon, second report to Organon). This result will now be examined more closely since it is susceptible to a pertinent explanation, as follows.

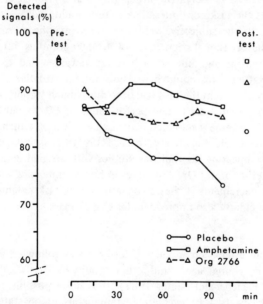

Fig. 7.3. Decrement across successive 15 minute periods of percentage signals detected under placebo compared with no decrement under dexamphetamine (10 mg) or polypeptide (Org 2766, 40 mg). Each active treatment compared with placebo: $p < 0.01$ (Newman–Keuls test). (Reproduced by kind permission of Dr J. F. O'Hanlon.)

A recent report by Parasuraman (1979) indicates that in successive-discrimination vigilance tasks (involving a memory load), as the task above, two types of vigilance decrement can occur. In terms of signal detection theory (not applied in the analyses of the above data) these decrements relate to two performance variables, described as d' and β. A decrement in sensitivity (d') over time occurs with a combination of poor-quality imput data (signal weak relative to 'noise'), poor representation of the stimulus characteristics in memory, and a high event rate. The resulting demand on perceptual processing can require too much attentional effort for sustained performance to be possible. Moreover, performance can be little improved by increasing the processing resources, since the limitations pertain to the signal-data and memory-data limits, i.e. to the task characteristics. This situation might have applied in the case of the elderly volunteers. The task parameters were deliberately set to maximize the occurrence of performance decrements (i.e. to produce a baseline level of 80–90 per cent correct responses) thereby making the task 'difficult'. Furthermore, these subjects are likely to have manifested minor visual and memory impairments together with slowness in central processing. Hence Org 2766 would not have reversed the decrement.

The alternative type of performance decrement relates to an increase in the response criterion (β) occurring as a function of time. In relatively 'easy' discriminations, sustained effort is not needed and d' remains stable over time, but subjects become more conservative in deciding that a given signal was a target, i.e. β increases as the task continues. The criterion adopted, i.e. the value of β, varies according to the subjective value put upon making a correct response. In such tasks, the occasional occurrence of a target stimulus during a long and boring vigil is reinforcing, but its subjective reward value diminishes with decreasing motivation. This could have been just the situation applying to the young volunteers. For them the task had been made much 'easier' (the parameters had been set to produce a baseline performance of 90–95 per cent correct). Accordingly their decrement reflected decreased motivation which Org 2766 was able to reverse, as it did together with ACTH/α-MSH$_{4-10}$ in Gaillard's studies. O'Hanlon is now repeating his vigilance studies with a signal detection analysis, to determine whether or not Org 2766 does in fact operate via d' or β in blocking the time-on-task decrement. If the effect resides in β, task parameters can then be set so that the elderly also improve under Org 2766.

Mood

A lack of reliable effects on mood self-rating scales following acute doses of either peptide, in young, aged, and other groups has been a general finding (Gaillard 1980; Pigache and Rigter 1981). It is quite possible that this arose because most scales used to evaluate instantaneous mood states, seem more sensitive to sedative than to activating drug effects.

Chronic dosing with Org 2766 (one to four weeks) was confined to the elderly, both healthy volunteers and patients. This choice was made at a stage when the peptide was expected to improve memory function. Although that hypothesis was not confirmed, effects attributable to improved mood were forthcoming. Of the four chronic dosing studies completed (double-blind and crossed-over in a total of 128 subjects), three yielded significant mood effects (Braverman *et al.* 1981; Ferris and Reisberg 1981; Willner 1981). The remaining study (Branconnier and Cole, report to Organon) probably failed, in the main, through having too few subjects (10) per treatment group. The scales used comprised self and observer mood ratings and ward behaviour ratings (for a detailed review see Pigache 1982). The results were consistent both within and between the studies and related to scale factors identified as: anxiety, depression, apathy/withdrawal, socialness, attention, and energy, all of which improved significantly under the peptide. Prospective studies are now under way using diagnostically more homogenous groups, and patients with sufficient pathology to make it clear whether or not the mood/behavioural changes produced by the peptide, have real clinical impact.

CONCLUSIONS

The study of structure and function in natural and synthetic ACTH/MSH peptides (Greven and De Wied 1973) resulting in the synthesis of Org 2766, appears to have produced a new category of alerting substances, lacking such effects as sympathetic stimulation, appetite suppression, sleep disturbance, or motor activation. The evidence in Man suggests that Org 2766 augments the fixation of attentional sets (selective attention) and also maintains vigilance, perhaps by enhancing motivation. The apparent effect on mood could be independent of the foregoing effects, or, as argued elsewhere (Pigache 1982), might be secondary to the postulated increase in motivation. Low motivation, possibly resulting from a diminished response to positive reinforcement (rewards) together with low expectations, is a feature of depressions (Layne 1980). It might be that Org 2766 and similar peptides increase motivation by amplifying the effects of positive reinforcement (Bohus 1981; De Kloet and De Wied 1980). Moreover, such an action would highlight relevant stimuli and so bears on selective attention. The anatomical location of the Pro-OMC pathways, the regional pattern of Org 2766 uptake in the brain, and the sites at which the peptide enhances cerebral glucose metabolism, suggest an overlap with Routtenberg's 'Arousal System II' mediated via the limbic system (in particular, septum and hippocampus) and controlling responses through incentive, i.e. reward, related stimuli (Routtenberg 1968).

At a more empirical level, and setting the above speculations aside, the profile of activity for Org 2766 could represent a useful adjunct in treating certain conditions in the elderly. If Org 2766 proves to have clinically significant anti-depressant effects, with improved vigilance and an enhanced fixation of attention, it could benefit many depressed and/or demented patients. This is even more so, since it lacks sedative, anticholinergic, and, at present, any other side-effects. The incidence of depression is high in the elderly, with symptoms also present in 50 per cent of a mixed group of dements (Gottfries 1981). Depression is more heterogenous in the old than in the young (Blumenthal 1971), hence it could be, too, that a subgroup of patients exists who would respond selectively to the peptide. These mood effects were first seen in the elderly; thus the next stage of investigation continues in this age group, where more results are eagerly awaited. However, there is no reason to suppose that younger subjects are unresponsive to the peptide (witness for example the effects on vigilance) hence a question-mark appears in the title to this chapter. None the less, it does seem likely that there would be more indications for such a treatment in aged patients.

Acknowledgements

The author would like to thank many of his colleagues for their constructive criticism, especially Drs H. Greven and J. Paanakker, and Miss K. Mimpen for her patience.

REFERENCES

Akil. H. and Watson, S. J. (1980). Neuromodulatory functions of the brain pro-opiocortin system. In *Neural peptides and neuronal communication* (ed. E. Costa and M. Trabbuchi) pp. 435–45. Raven Press, New York.

Allen, J. P., Kendall, J. W., McGilvra, R., and Vincura, C. (1974). Immuno-reactive ACTH in cerebrospinal fluid. *J. clin. Endocr. Metab.* 38, 586–93.

Aronin, N. and Krieger, D. T. (1981). Measurement of ACTH and lipotropins. In *Frontiers of hormone research, ACTH and LPH in health and disease* (ed. Tj. B. Van Wimersma Greidanus and L. H. Rees) Vol. 8, pp. 62–79. Karger, Basel.

Ball, M. J. (1977). Neuronal loss, neurofibrillary tangles and granulovacuolar degeneration in the hippocampus with ageing and dementia. *Acta neuropath.* 37, 111–18.

Beckwith, B. E. and Sandman, C. A. (1978). Behavioural influences of the neuropeptides ACTH and MSH: a methodological review. *Neurosci. behav. Rev.* 2, 311–38.

Beloff-Chain, A., Edwardson, J. A., and Hawthorn, J. (1977). Corticotrophin-like intermediate lobe peptide as an insulin secretagogue. *Proc. Soc. Endocr.* 73, 28–9P.

Bergland, R. M. and Page, R. B. (1978). Can the pituitary secrete directly to the brain? (Affirmative anatomical evidence.) *Endocrinology* 102, 1325–38.

—— —— (1979). Pituitary-brain vascular relations: a new paradigm. *Science, NY* 204, 18–24.

Besser, G. M. (1981). Adrenocorticotrophin and lipotrophin in pituitary–adreno-cortical disease. In *Frontiers of hormone research, ACTH and LPH in health and disease* (ed. Tj. B. Van Wimersma Greidanus and L. H. Rees) Vol. 8, pp. 80–106. Karger, Basel.

Bijlsma, W. A., Jennekens, F. G. I., Schotman, P., and Gispen, W. H. (1981). Effects of corticotrophin (ACTH) on peripheral nerve regeneration: structure–activity study. *Eur. J. Pharmac.* 70, 73–9.

Bloom, F. E. and Hendriksen, S. J. (1982). Endorphin studies: electrophysiologic and behavioural effects. In *Modern problems of pharmacopsychiatry. The role of endorphins in neuropsychiatry* (ed. H. M. Emrich) Vol. 17, pp. 19–37. Karger, Basel.

Blumenthal, M. D. (1974). Heterogeneity and research on depressive disorders. *Archs. gen. Psychiat.* 24, 524–31.

Bohus, B. (1981). Neuropeptides in brain functions and dysfunctions. *Int. J. ment. Hlth* 9, 6–44.

—— and De Kloet, E. R. (1979). Behavioural effects of neuropeptides (endorphins, enkephalins, ACTH fragments) and corticosteroids. In *Interaction within the brain-pituitary-adrenocortical system* (ed. M. T. Jones, B. Gillham, M. F. Dallman, and S. Chattopadhyay) pp. 7–16. Academic Press, London.

—— and De Wied, D. (1967). Failure of α-MSH to delay extinction of conditioned behaviour in rats with lesions of the parafascicular nucleus of the thalamus *Physiol. Behav.* 2, 221–3.

—— —— (1980). Pituitary-adrenal system hormones and adaptive behaviour. In *General, comparative and clinical endocrinology of the adrenal cortex*, Vol. 3 (ed. I. C. Jones and I. W. Henderson) pp. 265–347. Academic Press, London

Branconnier, R. J., Cole, J. O., and Gardos, G. (1979). ACTH$_{4-10}$ in the amelior ation of neuropsychological symptomatology associated with senile organic brain syndrome. *Psychopharmacology* 61, 161–5.

Braverman, A., Hamdy, R., Meisner, P., and Perera, N. (1981). Clinical trial of Org 2766 (ACTH$_{4-9}$ analogue) in the treatment of elderly people with impaired function. Paper presented at the *III World Congress of Biological Psychiatry*, Stockholm, 28 June–3 July.

Breier, C., Kain, H., and Konzett, H. (1979). Personality dependent effect of the ACTH$_{4-10}$ fragment on test performances and on concomitant autonomic reactions. *Psychopharmacology* **65**, 239–45.

Brownstein, M. J. (1980). Adrenocorticotropic hormone (ACTH) in the central nervous system. In *Neural peptides and neuronal communication* (ed. E. Costa and M. Trabbucchi) pp. 93–9. Raven Press, New York.

Brunia, C. H. M. and Van Boxtel, A. (1978). MSH/ACTH$_{4-10}$ and task-induced increase in tendon reflexes and heart rate. *Pharmac. Biochem. Behav.* **9**, 615–18;

Burbach, J. P. H., Loeber, J. G., Verhoef, J., Wiegant, V. M., De Kloet, E. R., and De Wied, D. (1980). Selective conversion of β-endorphin into peptides related to γ- and α-endorphin. *Nature, Lond.* **283**, 96–7.

Celio, M. R., Höllt, V., Buetti, G., Pasi, A., Bürginer, E., Eberle, A., Kopp, G., Siebenmann, R., Friede, R. L., Landolt, A., Binz, H., and Zenker, W. (1980). Immunohistochemical study of β-endorphin and related peptides in the 'invading cells' of the human neurohypophysis during ontogenesis and adulthood. In *Neural peptides and neuronal mechanisms* (ed. E. Costa and M. Trabbucchi) pp. 1–23. Raven Press, New York.

Challis, J. R. and Tarosis, J. D. (1977). Is alpha-MSH a trophic hormone to adrenal functions in the foetus? *Nature, Lond.* **269**, 818–19.

Chrétien, M., Seidah, N. G., Benjannet, S., Drâgon, N., Routhier, R., Motomatsu, T., Crine, P., and Lis, M. (1977). A β-LPH precursor model: recent developments concerning morphine-like substances. *Ann NY Acad. Sci.* **297**, 84–102.

Christensen, C. W., Hartson, C. T., Kastin, A. J., Kostrgzewa, R. M., and Spirtes, M. A. (1976). Preliminary investigation on α-MSH and MIF 1 effects on cyclic AMP levels in rat brain. *Pharmac. Biochem. Behav.* **5**, Suppl. 1, 117–20.

Daly, J. (1977). *Cyclic nucleotides in the nervous system*, pp. 11. Plenum Press, New York.

De Kloet, E. R. and De Wied, D. (1980). The brain as target tissue for hormones of pituitary origin: behavioural and biochemical studies. In *Frontiers of neuroendocrinology* (Ed. L. Martini and W. F. Ganong) Vol. 6, pp. 157–201. Raven Press, New York.

— Veldhuis, D., and Bohus, B. (1980). Significance of neuropeptides in the control of corticosterone receptor activity in rat brain. In *Receptors for neurotransmitters and peptides hormones* (ed. G. Pepeu, M. J. Kuhar, and S. J. Enna) pp. 373–82. Raven Press, New York.

— Wallach, G., and McEwen, B. S. (1975). Differences in corticosterone and dexamethasone binding to rat brain and pituitary. *Endocrinology* **96**, 598–609.

Delanoy, R. L. and Dunn, A. J. (1978). Mouse brain deoxyglucose uptake after footshock, ACTH analogs, α-MSH, corticosterone or lysine vasopressin. *Pharmac. Biochem. Behav.* **9**, 21–6.

De Vellis, J. and Kukes, G. (1973). Regulation of glial cell functions by hormones and ions: a review. *Texas Rep. Biol. Med.* **31**, 271–93.

De Wied, D., Bohus, B., Van Ree, J. M., and Urban, I. (1978). Behavioural and electrophysiological effects of peptides related to lipotropin (β-LPH). *J. Pharmac. exp. Ther.* **204**, 570–80.

— Witter, A., and Greven, H. M. (1975). Behaviourally active ACTH analogues. *Biochem. Pharmac.* **24**, 1463–8.

Dunn, A. J. and Gispen, W. H. (1977). How ACTH acts on the brain. *Biobehav. Rev.* **1**, 15–23.

Eckman, W. W., Phair, R. D., Fernstermacher, J. D., Patlak, C. S., Kennedy, C., and Sokoloff, L. (1975). Permeability limitation in estimation of local brain blood flow with ^{14}C-antipyrene. *Am. J. Physiol.* **229**, 215–21.

Eklöff, B., Lassen, N. A., Nilsson, L., Norberg, K., Siesjö, B. K., and Torlöf, P. (1974). Regional cerebral blood flow in the rat measured by the tissue sampling technique; a critical evaluation using four indicators ^{14}C-antipyrene, ^{14}C-ethanol, ^{3}H-water, and ^{133}xenon. *Acta physiol. Scand.* **91**, 1–10.

Endroczi, E., Lissak, K., Fekete, T., and De Wied, D. (1970). Effects of ACTH on EEG habituation in human subjects. *Prog. Brain Res.* **32**, 254–62.

Fehm-Wolfsdorf, G., Elbert, T., Lutzenberger, W., Rockstroh, B., Birbaumer, N., and Fehm, H. L. (1981). Effects of ACTH$_{4-9}$ analog on human cortical evoked potentials in a two-stimulus reaction time paradigm. *Psychoneuroendocrinology*, **6**, 311–19.

Ferris, S. H. and Reisberg, B. (1981). Clinical studies of neuropeptide treatment in impaired elderly. Paper presented at the *III World Congress of Biological Psychiatry*, Stockholm, 28 June–3 July.

Gaillard, A. W. K. (in press). ACTH analogues and human performance. In *Endogenous peptides and learning and memory processes* (ed. J. L. Martinez, R. A. Jensen, R. B. Messing, H. Rigter, and J. L. McGaugh). Academic Press, New York.

—— and Sanders, A. F. (1975). Some effects of ACTH$_{4-10}$ on performance during a serial reaction task. *Psychopharmacologia* **42**, 201–8.

—— and Varey, C. A. (1979). Some effects of an ACTH$_{4-9}$ analog (Org 2766) on human performance. *Physiol. Behav.* **23**, 78–84.

Gann, D. S., Ward, D. G., and Carlson, D. E. (1979). Neural pathways controlling release of corticotrophin (ACTH). In *Interaction within the brain–pituitary–adrenocortical system* (ed. M. J. Jones, B. Gillham, M. F. Dallman, and S. Chattopadhyay) pp. 75–86. Academic Press, London.

Gispen, W. H., Reigth, M. E. A., Schotman, P., Wiegant, V. M., Zwiers, H., and De Wied, D. (1977). CNS and ACTH-like peptides: neurochemical response and interaction with opiates. In *Neuropeptide influence on the brain and behaviour* (eds. L. H. Miller, C. A. Sandman, and A. J. Kastin) pp. 61–80. Raven Press, New York.

—— Wiegant, V M., Greven, H. M., and De Wied, D. (1975). The induction of excessive grooming in the rat by intraventricular application of peptides derived from ACTH: structure–activity studies. *Life Sci.* **17**, 645–52.

Goldman, H., Murphy, S., Schneider, D. R., and Felt, B. T. (1979). Cerebral blood flow after treatment with Org 2766, a potent analog of ACTH$_{4-9}$. *Pharmac. Biochem. Behav.* **10**, 883–7.

—— Sandman, C. A., Kastin, A., and Murphy, S. (1975). MSH affects regional perfusion of the brain. *Pharmac. Biochem. Behav.* **3**, 661–4.

Gottfries, C. G. (1981). Treatment of depression in the elderly. General clinical considerations. *Acta psychiat. scand.* **63**, Suppl. 290, 401–9.

Greenberg, R., Whalley, C. E., Jourdikian, F., Mendelson, I. S., Walter, R., Nikolics, K., Coy, D. H., Schally, A. V., and Kastin, A. J. (1976). Peptides readily penetrate the blood-brain barrier: uptake of peptides by synaptosomes is passive. *Pharmac. Biochem. Behav.* **5**, Suppl. 1, 151–8.

Greven, H. M. and De Wied, D. (1973). The influence of peptides derived from corticotrophin (ACTH) on performance. Structure activity studies. In *Progress in brain research, drug effects on neuroendocrine regulation* (ed. E. Zimmerman, W. H. Gispen, B. H. Marks, and D. De Wied) Vol. 39, pp. 429–42. Elsevier, Amsterdam.

—— —— (1977). Influence of peptides structurally related to ACTH and MSH on active avoidance behaviour in rats. In *Frontiers of hormone research* (ed. Tj. B. Van Wimersma Greidanus) pp. 140–52. Karger, Basel.

—— —— (1980). Structure and behavioural activity of peptides related to cortico-

trophin and lipotrophin. In *Hormones and the brain* (eds. D. De Wied and
P. A. Van Keep) pp. 115–27. MTP Press, Lancaster.
Hillyard, S. A., Picton, T. W., and Regan, D. (1978). Sensation, perception and
attention: analysis using ERPs. In *Event-related brain potentials in man*
(ed. E. Callaway, P. Tueting, and S. Koslow) pp. 223–322. Academic Press,
New York.
Hökfelt, T., Lundberg, J. M., Schultzberg, M., Johansson, O., Ljungdahl, A., and
Rehfeld, J. (1980). Coexistence of peptides and putative transmitters in
neurones. In *Neural peptides and neuronal communication* (ed. E. Costa
and M. Trabbucchi) pp. 1–23. Raven Press, New York.
Hope, J. and Lowry, P. J. (1981). Pro-opiocortin: the ACTH/LPH common
precursor protein. In *Frontiers of hormone research, ACTH and LPH in
health and disease* (ed. Tj. B. Van Wimersma Greidanus and L. H. Rees)
Vol. 8, pp. 44–61. Karger, Basel.
Hosobuchi, Y. (1982). Periaqueductal gray stimulation in humans produces
analgesia accompanied by elevation of β-endorphin and ACTH in ventricular
CSF. In *Modern problems of pharmacopsychiatry. The role of endorphins
in neuropsychiatry* (ed. H. M. Emrich) Vol. 17, pp. 109–22. Karger, Basel.
Jacquet, Y.-F. (1978). Opiate effects after adrenocorticotropin or β-endorphin
injection into the periaqueductal gray matter of rats. *Science, NY* **201**,
1032–4.
Jordan, R. M., Kendall, J. W., Seaich, J. L., Allen, J. P., Paulsen, C. A., Kerber,
C. W., and Vanderlaan, W. P. (1976). Cerebrospinal fluid hormone concentration in the evaluation of pituitary tumours. *Ann. intern. Med.* **85**, 49–95.
Kendall, J. and Orwoll, E. (1980). Anterior pituitary hormones in the brain and
other extrapituitary sites. In *Frontiers in neuroendocrinology* (ed. L. Martini
and W. F. Ganong) Vol. 6, pp. 33–65. Raven Press, New York.
King, A. C. and Cuatrescasas, P. (1981). Peptide hormone-induced receptor
mobility, aggregation and internalization. *New Engl. J. Med.* **305**, 77–88.
Kleber, G., Gramsch, C., Höllt, V., Mehraein, P., Pasi, A., and Herz, A. (1980).
Extrahypothalamic corticotropin and α-melanotropin in human brain. *Neuroendocrinology* **31**, 39–45.
Knigge, K. M., Joseph, S. A., Silverman, A. J., and Vaala, S. (1973). Further
observations on the structure and function of the median eminence with
reference to the organisation of RF-producing elements in the endocrine
hypothalamus. *Prog. Brain Res.* **39**, 7–20.
Knizely, H. (1972). The hippocampus and septal area as primary target sites for
corticosterone. *J. Neurochem.* **19**, 2737–45.
Krieger, D. T. and Liotta, A. S. (1979). Pituitary hormones in the brain: where,
how and why? *Science, NY* **205**, 266–72.
— — and Brownstein, M. J. (1977a). Presence of corticotropin in brain of
normal and hypophysectomized rats. *Proc. natn. Acad. Sci. USA* **74**, 648–52.
— — — (1977b). Presence of corticotropin in limbic system of normal and
hypophysectomized rats. *Brain Res.* **128**, 575–9.
— and Martin, J. B. (1981). Brain peptides. *New Engl. J. Med.* **304**, 876–85.
Landfield, P. W., Baskin, R. K., and Pitler, T. A. (1981). Brain aging correlates:
retardation by hormonal–pharmacological treatments. *Science, NY* **214**,
581–4.
— Lindsey, J. D., and Lynch, G. (1978a). Apparent acceleration of brain aging
pathology by prolonged administration of glucocorticoids. *Soc. Neurosci. Abstr.*
4, 350.
— Rose, G., Sandles, L., Wohlstadter, T., and Lynch, G. (1977). Patterns of
astroglial hypertrophy and neuronal degeneration in the hippocampus of
aged, memory-deficient rats. *Gerontology* **32**, 3–12.
— Waymire, J. C., and Lynch, G. (1978b). Hippocampal aging and adreno-

corticoids: quantitative correlations. *Science, NY* **202**, 1098-102.
— Wurtz, C., Lindsey, J. D., and Lynch, G. (1979). Long-term adrenalectomy reduces some morphological correlates of brain aging. *Soc. Neurosci. Abstr.* **5**, 20.
Larsson, L.-I. (1977). Corticotropin-like peptides in central nerves and in endocrine cells of gut and pancreas. *Lancet* 1321-3.
— (1980). Corticotropin and α-melanotropin in brain nerves: immunocytochemical evidence for axonal transport and processing. In *Neural peptides and neuronal communication* (ed. E. Costa and M. Trabbucchi) pp. 101-7. Raven Press, New York.
Layne, C. (1980). Motivational deficit in depression: people's expectation x outcomes' impact. *J. clin. Psychol.* **36**, 647-52.
Li, C. H., Yamashiro, D., Chung, D., Doneen, B. A., Loh, H. H., and Tseng, L.-f. (1977). Isolation, structure, synthesis and morphine-like activity of β-endorphin from human pituitary glands. *Ann. NY Acad. Sci.* **297**, 158-66.
Lichtensteiger, W. and Monnet, F. (1979). Differential response of dopamine neurons to α-melanotropin and analogues in relation to their endocrine and behavioural potency. *Life Sci.* **25**, 2079-87.
Lindsey, J. D., Landfield, P. W., and Lynch, G. (1979). Early onset and topographical distribution of hypertrophied astrocytes in hippocampus of aging rats. *J. Geront.* **23**, 661-71.
Lovejoy, E. (1966). Analysis of the overlearning reversal effect. *Psychol. Rev.* **73**, 86-103.
Lowry, P. J. and Rees, L. H. (1978). Corticotropin-like peptides outside the pituitary. *Lancet* 273.
— Silman, R. E., Hope, J., and Scott, A. P. (1977). Structure and biosynthesis of peptides related to corticotropins and β-melanotropins. *Ann. NY Acad. Sci.* **297**, 49-62.
McCarthy, G. and Donchin, E. (1981). A metric for thought: a comparison of P 300 latency and reaction time. *Science NY* **211**, 77-80.
McCulloch, J., Kelly, P. A. T., and Van Delft, A. M. L. (1981). Neuroanatomical basis for the action of a behaviourally active ACTH$_{4-9}$ analog. *Eur. J. Pharmac.* in press.
McEwen, B. S., De Kloet, R., and Wallach, G. (1976). Interaction *in vivo* and *in vitro* of corticoids and progesterone with cell nuclei and soluble macromolecules from rat brain regions and pituitary. *Brain Res.* **105**, 129-36.
— Gerlach, J. L., and Micco, D. J. (1975). Putative glucocorticoid receptors in hippocampus and other regions of the rat brain. In *The hippocampus*, Vol. 1 (ed. R. L. Isaacson and K. H. Pribram) pp. 285-322. Plenum Press, New York.
— Zigmond, R. E., and Gerlach, J. L. (1972). Sites of steroid binding and action in the brain. In *Structure and function of nervous tissue*, Vol. 5 (ed. H. Bourne) pp. 205-91. Academic Press, New York.
McLoughlin, L., Lowry, P. J., Rutter, S., Besser, G. M., and Rees, L. H. (1980). β-Endorphin and β-MSH in human plasma. *Clin. Endocr.* **12**, 287-92.
Mains, R. E., Eipper, B. A., and Ling, N. (1977). Common precursor to corticotropins and endorphins. *Proc. natn. Acad. Sci. USA* **74**, 3014-18.
Mezey, E., Kivovics, P., and Palkovits, M. (1979). Pituitary-brain retrograde transport. *Trends Neurosci.* **2**, 57-60.
— Palkovits, M., De Kloet, E. R., Verhoef, J. and De Wied, D. (1978). Evidence for pituitary-brain transport of a behaviourally potent ACTH analog. *Life Sci.* **22**, 831-8.
Miller, L. H., Harris, L. C., Van Riezen, H., and Kastin, A. J. (1976). Neuroheptapeptide influence on attention and memory in man. *Pharmac. Biochem. Behav.* **5**, Suppl. 1, 17-21.
— Kastin, A. J., Sandman, C. A., Fink, M., and Van Veen, W. (1974). Poly

peptide influences on attention, memory and anxiety in man. *Pharmac. Biochem. Behav.* **2**, 663-8.

Nakanishi, S., Inove, A., Kita, T., Nakamura, M., Chang, A., Cohen, S., and Numa, S. (1979). Nucleotide sequence of cloned c DNA for bovine corticotropin-β-lipotropin precursor. *Nature, Lond.* **278**, 423-7.

Nicholson, A. N. and Stone, B. M. (1980). A synthetic ACTH$_{4-9}$ analogue (Organon 2766) and sleep in healthy man. *Neuropharmacology* **15**, 1245-6.

Oliver, C., Mical, R. S., and Porter, J. C. (1977). Hypothalamic-pituitary vasculature — evidence for retrograde flow in the pituitary stalk. *Endocrinology* **101**, 598-604.

Palkovits, M. and Mezey, E. (1981). Anatomical connections between brain and anterior pituitary. In *Frontiers of hormone research, ACTH and LPH in health and disease* (ed. Tj. B. Van Wimersma Greidanus and L. H. Rees) Vol. 8, pp. 122-38. Karger, Basel.

Parasuraman, P. (1979). Memory load and event rate control sensitivity decrements in sustained attention. *Science, NY* **205**, 924-7.

— and Beatty, (1980). Brain events underlying detection and recognition of weak sensory signals. *Science, NY* **210**, 80-3.

Pelletier, G., Labrie, F., Kastin, A. J., Coy, D., and Schally, A. V. (1975). Radioautographic localisation of radioactivity in rat brain after intraventricular or intracarotid injection of ^{3}H-L-prolyl-L-leucyl glycinamide. *Pharmac. Biochem. Behav.* **3**, 675-9.

— Leclerc, R., Labrie, F., Cote, J., Chrétien, M., and Lis, M. (1977). Immunohistochemical localization of β-lipotrophin hormone in the pituitary gland. *Endocrinology* **100**, 770-6.

Peng Loh, Y. and Gainer, H. (1977). Heterogeneity of melanotropic peptides in the pars intermedia and brain. *Brain Res.* **130**, 169-75.

Pigache, R. M. (1982). Effects of ACTH-like peptides on cognition and affect in the elderly. In *Neuropeptides and hormone modulation of brain function and homeostasis* (ed. J. M. Ordy, J. R. Sladek, and B. Reisberg). Raven Press, New York.

— and Rigter, H. (1981). Effects of peptides related to ACTH on mood and vigilance in man. In *Frontiers of hormone research, ACTH and LPH in health and disease* (ed. Tj. B. Van Wimersma Greidanus and L. H. Rees) Vol. 8, pp. 193-207. Karger, Basel.

Rappoport, S. I. (1976). *Blood-brain barrier in physiology and medicine.* Raven Press, New York.

Rigter, H. and Crabbe, J. C. (1979). Modulation of memory by pituitary hormones and related peptides. *Vitam. Horm.* **37**, 153-241.

Roberts, J. L. and Herbert, E. (1977). Characterization of a common precursor to corticotropin and β-lipotropin: identification of β-lipotropin peptides and their arrangement relative to corticotropin in the precursor synthesized in a cell-free system. *Proc. natn. Acad. Sci. USA* **74**, 5300-4.

Rockstroh, B., Elbert, T., Lutzenberger, W., Birbaumer, N., Fehm, H. L., and Voigt, K.-H. (1981). Effects of an ACTH$_{4-9}$ analog on human cortical evoked potentials in a constant foreperiod reaction time paradigm. *Psychoneuroendocrinology* in press.

Routtenberg, A. (1968). The two-arousal hypothesis: reticular formation and limbic system. *Psychol. Rev.* **75**, 51-80.

Rudman, D. and Isaacs, J. W. (1975). Effects of intrathecal injection of melanotropic-lipolytic peptides on the concentration of $3', 5'$-cyclic adenosine monophosphate in cerebrospinal fluid. *Endocrinology* **97**, 1476-80.

Sakurada, O., Kennedy, C., Jehle, J., Brown, J. D., Carbin, G. W., and Sokoloff, L. (1978). Measurement of local cerebral blood flow with iodo-[^{14}C]-antipyrene. *Am. J. Physiol.* **234**, H 59-66.

94   *A peptide for the aged? Basic and clinical studies*

Sandman, C. A., Berka, C., Walker, B. B., and Veith, J. (in press). Dose relationships of a long acting analog of $ACTH_{4-9}$ on the human visual evoked response. *Psychopharmacology.*
—— George, J., McCanne, T. R., Nolan, J. D., Kaswan, J., and Kastin, A. J. (1977); $ASH/ACTH_{4-10}$ influences behavioural and physiological measures of attention. *J. clin. Endocr. Metab.* 44, 884–91.
—— —— Nolan, J. D., Van Riezen, H., and Kastin, A. J. (1975). Enhancement of attention in man with $ACTH/MSH_{4-10}$. *Physiol. Behav.* 15, 427–31.
—— —— Walker, B. B., Nolan, J. D., and Kastin, A. J. (1976). Neuropeptide $MSH/ACTH_{4-10}$ enhances attention in the mentally retarded. *Pharmac. Biochem. Behav.* 5, 23–8.
Schneider, D. R., Felt, B. T., and Goldman, H. (1977). Induction of brain cyclic AMP by $ACTH_{4-9}$ analogue. *Neuropharmacology* Abstr. 154.
—— —— Murphy, S., and Goldman, H. (1981a). Cyclic AMP in female mouse brain is altered by the adrenocorticotrophic hormone (4–9) analogue Organon 2766. *J. Neurochem.* 37, 537–42.
Schneider, E., Jacobi, P., Van Riezen, H., Voerman, J. W. A., and Fischer, P. A. (1981b). Wirkungen synthetischer Neuropeptide auf die hirnorganischen Leistungsinsuffizienz. Ergebnisse der Anwendung von $ACTH_{4-10}$ und des $ACTH_{4-9}$-Anologon. *Pharmacopsychiatrie* 14, 155–9.
Schwandt, P. (1981). Lypolytic effects of ACTH and lipotrophins. In *Frontiers of hormone research, ACTH and LPH in health and disease* (ed. Tj. B. Van Wimersma Greidanus and L. H. Rees) Vol. 8, pp. 107–21. Karger, Basel.
Shapiro, M. S., Namba, T., and Grob, D. (1968). The effect of corticotropin on the neuromuscular junction. Morphological studies in rabbits. *Neurology, Minneap.* 18, 1018–22.
Strand, F. L., Cayer, A., Gonzalez, E., and Stoboy, H. (1976). Peptide enhancement of neuromuscular function: animal and clinical studies. *Pharmac. Biochem. Behav.* 5, Suppl. 1, 179–87.
—— and Kung, T. T. (1980). ACTH accelerates recovery of neuromuscular function following crushing of peripheral nerve. *Peptides* 1, 135–8.
—— Stoboy, H., and Cayer, A. (1973/74). A possible direct action of ACTH on nerve and muscle. *Neuroendocrinology* 13, 1–20.
—— —— Friedebold, G., Krivoy, W., Heyck, H., and Van Riezen, H. (1977). Changes in muscle action potential in patients with diseases of motor units following the infusion of a peptide fragment of ACTH. *Arzneimittel.-Forsch.* 27, 681–3.
Stumpf, W. E. and Sar, M. (1975). Anatomical distribution of corticosterone-concentrating neurons in rat brain. In *Anatomical neuroendocrinology. Int. Conf. Neurobiology of CNS-hormone interactions*, pp. 254–61. Karger, Basel.
Sutherland, N. S. (1959). Stimulus analysing mechanisms. *Proc. Symp. on the Mechanization of Thought Processes*, Vol. 2, pp. 575–609. HMSO, London.
Swanson, L. H. and Cowan, W. M. (1977). An autoradiographic study of the organisation of the efferent connections of the hippocampal formation in the rat. *J. comp. Neurol.* 172, 49–84.
Tighe, T. J., Glick, J., and Cole, M. (1971). Subproblem analysis of discrimination shift learning. *Psychon. Sci.* 24, 159–60.
Thody, A. J. (1977). The significance of melanocyte stimulating hormone (MSH) and the control of its secretion in the mammal. In *Advances in drug research* (ed. Harper and Simmonds) Vol. 2, pp. 23–74. Academic Press, London.
Tomlinson, B. E. and Henderson, G. (1976). Some quantitative cerebral findings in normal and demented old people. In *Neurobiology of aging* (ed. R. D. Terry and S. Gershon) pp. 183–204. Raven Press, New York.
Urban, I. and De Wied, D. (1976). Changes in excitability of the theta activity generating substrate by $ACTH_{4-10}$ in the rat. *Exp. brain Res.* 24, 325–34.

Valero, I., Stewart, J., McNaughton, N., and Gray, J. A. (1977). Septal driving of the hippocampal theta rhythm as a function of frequency in the male rat: effects of adreno-pituitary hormones. *Neuroendocrinology* 2, 1029-32.
Van Nispen, J. W. and Greven, H. M. (1982). Structure-activity relationships of peptides derived from ACTH, β-LPH and MSH with regard to avoidance behaviour in rats. *Pharmac. Ther.* in press.
Van Ree, J. M. and De Wied, D. (1981). Behavioural effects of β-endorphin fragments. In *Frontiers of hormone research, ACTH and LPH in health and disease* (ed. Tj. B. Van Wimersma Greidanus and L. H. Rees) Vol. 8, pp. 178-92. Karger, Basel.
Van Wimersma Greidanus, Tj. B., Van Dijk, A. M. A., De Rotte, A. A., Goedemans, J. H. J., Croiset, G., and Thody, A. J. (1978). Involvement of ACTH and MSH in active and passive avoidance behaviour. *Brain Res. Bull.* 3, 227-30.
Vaudry, H., Tonon, M. C., Delarue, C., Vaillant, R., and Kraicer, J. (1978). Biological and radioimmunological evidence for melanocyte stimulating hormones (MSH) of extrapituitary origin in the rat brain. *Neuroendocrinology* 27, 9-24.
Verhoef, J., Palkovits, M., and Witter, A. (1977a). Distribution of a behaviourally highly potent ACTH₄₋₉ analog in rat brain after intraventricular administration. *Brain Res.* 126, 89-104.
— and Witter, A. (1976). In vivo fate of a behaviourally active ACTH₄₋₉ analog in rats after systemic administration. *Pharmac. Biochem. Behav.* 4, 583-90.
— — and De Wied, D. (1977b). Specific uptake of a behaviourally potent [³H]-ACTH₄₋₉ analog in the septal area after intraventricular injection in rats. *Brain Res.* 131, 117-28.
Versteeg, D. H. G. (1980). Interaction of peptides related to ACTH, MSH and β-LPH with neurotransmitters in the brain. *Psychopharmacologia* 11, 535-57.
Visser, M. and Swaab, D. F. (1977). α-MSH in the human pituitary. In *Frontiers in hormone research*, Vol. 4, pp. 42-5. Karger, Basel.
Walker, B. and Sandman, C. A. (1979). Influences of an analog of the neuropeptide ACTH₄₋₉ on mentally retarded adults. *Am. J. Ment. Defic.* 83, 346-52.
Walker, J. M., Berntson, G. G., Sandman, C. A., Kastin, A. J., and Akil, H. (1981). Induction of analgesia by central administration of Org 2766, an analog of ACTH₄₋₉. *Eur. J. Pharmac.* 69, 71-9.
Watson, S. J. and Akil, H. (1980). On the multiplicity of active substances in single neurons: β-endorphin and α-melanocyte stimulating hormone as a model system. In *Hormones and the brain* (ed. D. De Wied and P. A. Van Keep) pp. 73-86. MTP Press, Lancaster.
— — (1981a). Anatomical and functional studies of ACTH and lipotropin in the central nervous system. In *Frontiers of hormone research, ACTH and LPH in health and disease* (ed. Tj. B. Van Wimersma Greidanus and L. H. Rees) Vol. 8, pp. 149-61. Karger, Basel.
— — (1981b). Opioid peptides and related substances: immunocytochemistry. In *Advances in biochemical psychopharmacology, neurosecretion and brain peptides* (ed. J. B. Martin, S. Reichlin, and K. L. Bick) Vol. 28, pp. 77-86. Raven Press, New York.
— Barchas, J. D., and Li, C. H. (1977). β-Lipotropin: localization of cells and axons in rat brain by immunocytochemistry. *Proc. natn. Acad. Sci. USA* 74, 5155-8.
— Richard, C. W., and Barchas, J. D. (1978). Adrenocorticotropin in rat brain: immunocytochemical localization in cells and axons. *Science, NY* 200, 1180-2.
Weber, E., Martin, R., and Voight, K. H. (1979). Corticotropin/β-endorphin precursor: concomitant storage of its fragments in the secretory granules of anterior pituitary corticotrophin/endorphin cells. *Life Sci.* 25, 1111-18.
Wexler, B. C. (1976). Comparative aspects of hyperadrenocorticism and aging.

In *Hypothalamus, pituitary and aging* (ed. A. V. Everitt and J. A. Burgess) pp. 333–61. Thomas, Springfield, Ill.

Wiegant, V. M., Cools, A., and Gispen, W. H. (1977*a*). ACTH-induced excessive grooming involves brain dopamine. *Eur. J. Pharmac.* 41, 343–5.

—— Dunn, A. J., Schotman, P., and Gispen, W. H. (1979). ACTH-like neurotropic peptides: possible regulators of rat brain cyclic AMP. *Brain Res.* 168, 565–84.

—— and Gispen, W. H. (1975). ACTH$_{1-10}$ and cyclic AMP in rat brain slices. *Abstr. 5th Int. ISN Meeting*, Barcelona, p. 205.

—— —— Terenius, L., and De Wied, D. (1977*b*). ACTH-like peptides and morphine: interaction at the level of the CNS. *Psychoneuro-endocrinology* 2, 63–9.

—— Zwiers, H., and Gispen, W. H. (1981). Neuropeptides and brain cAMP and phosphoproteins. *Pharmac. Ther.* 12, 463–90.

Will, J. C., Abuzzahab, F. S., and Zimmerman, R. L. (1978). The effects of ACTH$_{4-10}$ versus placebo in the memory of symptomatic geriatric volunteers. *Psychopharmac. Bull.* 14, 25–7.

Willner, A. E. (1981). Influence of an analog of ACTH$_{4-9}$ (Org 2766) on mood in elderly symptomatic volunteers. Paper presented at *III World Congress of Biological Psychiatry*, Stockholm, 28 June–3 July.

Wisniewski, H. M. and Terry, R. D. (1973). Morphology of the aging brain, human and animal. *Prog. Brain Res.* 40, 167–86.

Witter, A., Greven, H. M., and De Wied, D. (1975). Correlation between structure, behavioural activity and rate of biotransformation of some ACTH$_{4-9}$ analogs. *J. Pharmac. exp. Ther.* 193, 853–60.

Wood, P. L., Malthe-Sørenssen, D., Cheney, D. L., and Costa, E. (1978). Increase of hippocampal acetylcholine turnover rate and the stretching–yawning syndrome elicited by alpha-MSH and ACTH. *Life Sci.* 22, 673–8.

Zeaman, D. and House, B. J. (1963). The role of attention in retardate discrimination learning. In *Handbook of mental deficiency* (ed. N. R. Ellis) pp. 159–223. McGraw-Hill, New York.

8

A peptide for the aged? – Animal studies

HENK RIGTER

The foundations for the behavioural pharmacology of hypophyseal peptides, including ACTH, were laid in the 1950s and 1960s. Early studies suggested that ACTH-like peptides may play a role in neural processes mediating adaptive behaviour. An important research strategy was the study of behavioural deficits in hypophysectomized rats. The rationale was simple and effective. If ACTH released from the pituitary gland is involved in the mediation of adaptive behaviour, extirpation of this gland should lead to behavioural deficits which can be corrected by treatment with exogenous ACTH. The great advocate of this strategy was De Wied. He and his group performed pioneering studies which basically confirmed their hypothesis. In the 1960s, this group of investigators started to examine the ability of hypophysectomized rats to learn (acquire) and maintain a 'shuttlebox' response. The shuttlebox is a set-up in which an animal is given a warning signal shortly before the delivery of an aversive stimulus, a mild electric shock to the feet. Rats readily learn to respond to the warning signal by moving from one side of the shuttlebox to the other, thus avoiding the shock. Learning performance of hypophysectomized rats was impaired in this task, and could be restored by treatment with ACTH (De Wied 1969) and its fragment $ACTH_{4-10}$ (De Wied 1969; Bohus *et al.* 1973). $ACTH_{4-10}$ is a peptide which is virtually devoid of known peripheral endocrine activities (De Wied 1969).

The example of $ACTH_{4-10}$ suggests that the effects of ACTH-like peptides on peripheral endocrine processes are dissociated from their effects on behaviour. This has been confirmed by the demonstration that ACTH is behaviourally active in adrenalectomized rats; that the behavioural activity of ACTH-like peptides is dependent upon the integrity of a number of structures in the midbrain–limbic system; and that these peptides also influence behaviour when injected in very low doses into the cerebral ventricles (for reviews, cf. De Wied 1977; Rigter and Crabbe 1979).

ACTH AND BEHAVIOUR

Which aspect of adaptive behaviour is influenced by ACTH? Many functions are required for adequate performance of an animal in the shuttlebox test, e.g. perception, locomotion, motivation, attention, learning and memory. It is very difficult to experimentally 'dissect' these functions. It is still not completely clear which function(s) is (are) influenced by ACTH and related peptides. There is more certainty as to which functions are *not* affected by the peptide treatment.

Experimental evidence

$ACTH_{1-10}$, a fragment with the same behavioural activity as $ACTH_{4-10}$, did not restore the somewhat altered responsiveness of hypophysectomized rats to a pain stimulus (Gispen *et al.* 1970). $ACTH_{4-10}$ did not change locomotor behaviour of hypophysectomized rats, when tested in the shuttlebox in the absence of the warning signal and the electric shock (Bohus *et al.* 1973). There have been reports that ACTH and $ACTH_{4-10}$ may improve memory consolidation (Flood *et al.* 1976; Gold and McGaugh 1977) but the preponderance of the evidence suggests that this effect, especially for the ACTH-fragments, is weak at best (cf. Rigter and Crabbe 1979). At any rate, it is highly unlikely that the restorative effect of ACTH-like peptides on acquisition of the shuttlebox response by hypophysectomized rats is due to some action on memory processes.

This was nicely demonstrated by Bohus *et al.* (1973). Rats from which the pituitary gland had been removed were trained in the shuttlebox for 14 days. Placebo-treated rats never reached a performance level that was higher than 50 per cent (50 per cent correct, i.e. avoidance, responses for a particular day). The behavioural anomaly was virtually corrected by treatment with $ACTH_{4-10}$, treatment being restricted to the first week of the experiment. At the end of that week, $ACTH_{4-10}$-injected rats had attained a performance level of 80 per cent avoidance responses. This relatively high performance level suggests that the animals had adequately learned (memorized) relevant information. In the second week, the administration of the peptide was stopped and this resulted in a gradual decline of performance to the level of the control group (Fig. 8.1). If $ACTH_{4-10}$ had normalized memory consolidation, there is no apparent

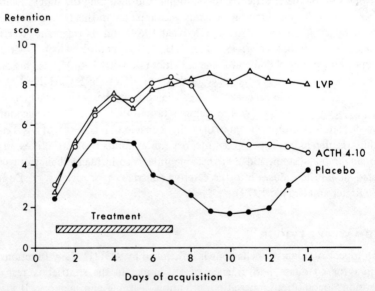

Fig. 8.1. The effect of $ACTH_{4-10}$ and vasopressin on deficient acquisition of a shuttlebox avoidance response in hypophysectomized male rats. In contrast to vasopressin, cessation of $ACTH_{4-10}$ treatment resulted in a decline in performance. (From Bohus *et al.* (1973), with kind permission.)

explanation why cessation of treatment after consolidation of memory had occurred should have produced a clear worsening of performance.

Basis of behavioural activity

Which explanations for the behavioural activity of ACTH-like peptides remain? There is general agreement that these peptides influence a process, or processes, akin to attention and motivation. Such an effect is probably not limited to hypophysectomized animals. In intact animals effects of ACTH and related peptides have been found which can be interpreted in similar terms. For example, ACTH-like peptides delay extinction of conditioned behaviour in intact rats. In the shuttlebox, and similar tests, extinction can be assessed when the warning signal is no longer followed by electric shock. When the animal (gradually) stops responding to the signal, one speaks of 'extinction' of conditioned behaviour. ACTH-like peptides caused animals to persevere in responding to the signal and thus delayed extinction (De Wied 1969; Greven and De Wied 1973). This effect of the peptides has not only been seen in tests involving extinction of fear-motivated responses, but also in tests of extinction of food- or sexually-motivated responses (Garrud et al. 1974; Bohus et al. 1975). Therefore, the influence of ACTH-like peptides is not confined to fear-motivation. However, ACTH, and some of its fragments and analogues, do not produce generalized changes in motivation. There is a clear element of specificity in the behavioural effects of this hormone (see previous chapter).

As mentioned above, the behavioural 'substrate' of ACTH seems to be a process, or processes, akin to attention and motivation. Attempts to specify this process are the refined motivation hypothesis proposed by De Wied (1977), which states that ACTH-like peptides enhance arousal in response to motivationally relevant cues, and the similar view expressed by Sandman and Kastin (1977), viz. that ACTH-like peptides facilitate 'selective' attention. The improvement of acquisition of the shuttlebox response by ACTH in hypophysectomized rats, and the delay of extinction in intact rats could be explained in this way. Two further examples will be given here, the first being taken from the work of Sandman and Kastin. These investigators have performed many experiments with α-MSH, which contains the first 13 amino-acids of ACTH with an acetyl group in front. α-MSH and ACTH have generally been found to exert similar behavioural effects. Thus, both peptides normalized deficient acquisition of the shuttlebox response in hypophysectomized rats (De Wied 1969) and delayed extinction of rewarded or punished responses (Garrud et al. 1974; Kastin et al. 1974; Rigter and Popping 1976). α-MSH also influenced reversal learning (Sandman et al. 1973). Rats were trained to select a white door rather than a black door, in order to escape or avoid electric shock. During subsequent reversal learning the rats were trained to choose the black door. Peptide-treated animals showed greater ease in mastering the reversal problem than the placebo-treated animals. It was suggested that the hormone had helped the rats during initial learning to pay attention to the essential cues of the task, including the black door.

The related motivation hypothesis is supported by data from self-stimulation experiments. Electrical stimulation of various brain areas is rewarding: animals with electrodes positioned in these areas learn to self-administer electrical stimulation, e.g. by pressing a bar. Org 2766 enhanced self-stimulation behaviour (Katz 1980) and a comparison between $ACTH_{4-10}$ and Org 2766 indicated that both peptides enhanced self-stimulation behaviour, but only when basal levels of responding were low. Org 2766 was a thousand times more potent than $ACTH_{4-10}$ (Fekete and De Wied 1981; and personal communication).

Structure–activity studies

Most structure–activity studies with ACTH have been performed by Greven and De Wied using the pole-jump extinction test (Greven and De Wied 1973, 1980). The pole-jump test, like the shuttlebox test, is an avoidance task. Rats were taught to associate a warning signal (a light) with impending electric shock to the feet. The animals could avoid the aversive stimulus by jumping on to a vertical pole (Fig. 8.2). The rats acquired the avoidance response in three days, and

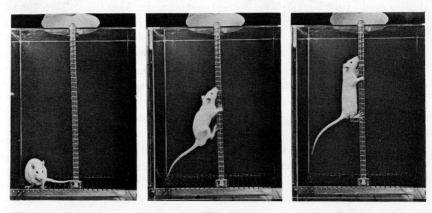

Fig. 8.2. Pole-jump avoidance test. The rat jumps onto the pole when the lamp on top of the box is lighted, in order to avoid the delivery of electric shock through the grid floor of the box.

extinction was assessed on the fourth day, peptide treatment being given 2–4 hours before the extinction tests. Several loci within the ACTH molecule were found to contribute to the effect of the hormone on extinction and $ACTH_{1-10}$ was almost as active as the full amino-acid sequence, $ACTH_{1-39}$ (Fig. 8.3). Step-by-step shortening, beginning at the N-terminus of the $ACTH_{1-10}$ fragment, indicated that $ACTH_{4-10}$ still had considerable behavioural activity. Shortening beginning at the C-terminus of the $ACTH_{1-10}$ fragment yielded $ACTH_{4-7}$ as the shortest sequence with clear-cut behavioural effect (Fig. 8.3). The peptides $ACTH_{7-10}$, $ACTH_{11-24}$, and $ACTH_{25-39}$ had one-tenth of the potency of $ACTH_{4-7}$. The residual potency of $ACTH_{7-10}$ could be enhanced to the level of the reference peptide 4–7 by extending the C-terminal sequence to $ACTH_{7-16}$-NH_2. Apparently, portions of the ACTH molecule other than the 4–7 sequence also possess some information for the behavioural activity in the pole-jump extinction test.

Through the introduction of modifications in the sequence $ACTH_{4-10}$ increases

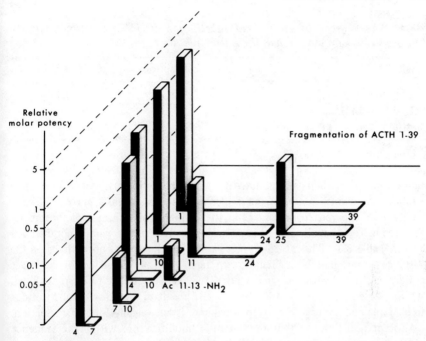

Fig. 8.3. Relative molar potencies of s.c. injected ACTH-fragments in the pole-jump extinction test. (Slightly modifed from Greven and De Wied (1980), with kind permission.)

in behavioural potency could be achieved. Oxidation of the methionine residue was very effective in this respect. This modification is known to reduce melanocyte-stimulating activity (see previous chapter); the enhanced behavioural potency produced by this structural change is therefore further evidence for the dissociation of behavioural and peripheral endocrine activities within the ACTH molecule. Peptides with methionine sulphoxide, $Met(O)^4$, and with methionine sulphone, $Met(O_2)^4$, did not differ much in behavioural activity. For practical reasons, the $Met(O_2)^4$ variant was selected for further attempts to increase the behavioural potency of ACTH-analogues. These attempts also included systematic substitutions by amino-acids in the D-configuration. Starting point was the sequence $ACTH_{4-9}$: H-Met-Glu-His-Phe-Arg-Trp-OH.

Replacement of Arg^8 by $D\text{-}Lys^8$ was most successful; this modification resulted in a 10–30 times more active compound. A further substitution, replacement of Trp^9 by Phe^9, slightly increased potency. The simultaneous introduction of the three modifications discussed yielded a peptide that was 1000 times as active as $ACTH_{4-9}$ in the pole-jump extinction test: H-Met(O_2)-Glu-His-Phe-D-Lys-Phe-OH. This peptide has been tentatively named Org 2766.

Potentiated activity of Org 2766

Witter *et al.* (1975) have tested the hypothesis that the potentiated activity of peptides like Org 2766 may be due to increased resistance against enzymatic degradation. ^{14}C-labelled $ACTH_{4-9}$-analogues were incubated with rat plasma or

TABLE 8.1.   *Effect of amino-acid substitution in $[^{14}C]$-ϵ-N-dimethyllysine (Lys*)-ACTH$_{4-9}$ on* in vitro *half-life (mean minutes ± s.e.m.)*

Peptide	Rat plasma	Rat brain extracts
[Lys^8*, Phe^9] ACTH$_{4-9}$	2.8 ± 0.6	< 1
[D-Lys^8*] ACTH$_{4-9}$	25 ± 3	4.5 ± 0.4
[Met(O)^4, D-Lys^8*, Phe^9] ACTH$_{4-9}$	74 ± 8	38 ± 3

From Witter *et al.* (1975).

brain extracts. The behavioural activity of all nine radioactive lysine-containing metabolic fragments ranged from 5 per cent to less than 1 per cent of the activity of the parent peptides. Thus, the biological significance of the metabolites seems to be small. The *in vitro* half-life values of the parent peptides are given in Table 8.1. The introduction of D-Lys^8 and Met(O)^4 both increased the resistance against metabolic breakdown. The *in vitro* half-life values of the intact peptides correlated with their behavioural activity. Witter *et al.* (1975) concluded that the increase in behavioural potency as a result of amino-acid substitutions can be explained, at least in part, by a higher resistance against biotransformation.

Another possibility is that the structural modifications within the sequence ACTH$_{4-9}$ have yielded a peptide with higher intrinsic activity and there are some structure–activity data that bear on this issue. For instance, the introduction of D-Lys in position 8 in ACTH$_{4-9}$ increased behavioural activity 10–30-fold; this is more than the threefold potentiation seen with D-Arg^8. These two peptides may be expected to have approximately the same resistance against metabolic degradation and so the higher potency of the D-Lys^8 peptide should be attributed to enhanced intrinsic activity (Greven and De Wied 1980).

It has been proposed that the pituitary gland or the brain may produce potent and specific behaviourally active peptides, which may be distinguished from ACTH and ACTH$_{4-10}$ (Loeber *et al.* 1979). Antibodies against Org 2766 were raised in rabbits and injected intracerebroventricularly into rats one hour before testing of pole-jump extinction. Cross-reactivity with ACTH and ACTH-fragments, such as the sequence 4–10, was very low (less than 0.1 per cent). The antibodies accelerated extinction and the investigators concluded that there may be hitherto unknown endogenous neuropeptide(s) involved in the mediation of adaptive behaviour. It is possible that Org 2766 resembles such endogenous peptides.

It is important to consider not only differences in potency but also differences in duration of action for various ACTH-fragments and analogues. A first study of the duration of action of Org 2766 was performed by Rigter *et al.* (1976). These investigators made use of the well-established phenomenon that ACTH-like peptides can attenuate experimentally-induced amnesia for a so-called passive avoidance response (cf. Rigter *et al.* 1974). The passive-avoidance apparatus consisted of a dark box with a small door, from which a narrow ledge protruded over empty space. A rat placed on such a ledge readily stepped into the box (Fig. 8.4) but when given an electric shock to the feet inside the box, it hesitated to re-enter the box when placed back on the ledge 24 hours later. The duration of

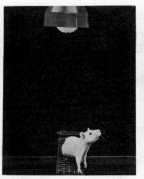 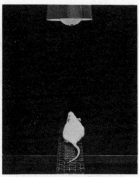 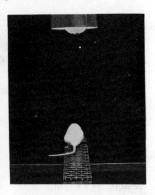

Fig. 8.4. The passive avoidance step-through task. A rat placed on the illuminated ledge will quickly enter the dark box. The animal will avoid entering the box when it has experienced a mild electric shock in the box on a previous occasion.

hesitation was taken as a measure of learned passive avoidance behaviour. Amnesia can be induced by a variety of treatments and the agent selected for the experiments of Rigter *et al.* (1976) was carbon dioxide (CO_2). Anaesthetizing rats with CO_2, immediately after delivery of the electric shock, resulted in amnesia. Rats thus treated usually re-entered the dark box almost as quickly as they used to do before the delivery of electric shock. Subcutaneous administration of ACTH-like peptides shortly before the retention test attenuated the amnesia. As in the pole-jump extinction test, Org 2766 was much more potent than $ACTH_{4-10}$; Org 2766 was also orally active. In a time-course study, a 100 μg/rat s.c. dose of $ACTH_{4-10}$ was effective when given within eight hours of the retention test and a similar duration of action was found for a 0.1 μg/rat s.c. dose of Org 2766.

With a change in behavioural paradigm, differences in duration of action for Org 2766 and $ACTH_{4-10}$ were detected by another group of investigators (Fekete and De Wied 1981; and personal communication). ACTH-like peptides enhanced performance of rats during testing of retention of a weak passive avoidance response. In these experiments, no amnesic treatment was given; rather the intensity of the electric shock was reduced so that avoidance behaviour of control rats was minimal. Under these conditions, Org 2766 (0.09 μg/rat s.c.) had a duration of action of approximately 24 hours, while the effect of $ACTH_{4-10}$ lasted 3-6 hours and was a 1000 times less potent. This long-lasting activity and the increase in potency for Org 2766 suggests that, in addition to enhanced resistance to biotransformation, enhanced intrinsic activity also plays a role in the effects of this peptide.

ORG 2766 IN THE BRAIN

Radioactive experiments

The studies by Verhoef have already been referred to in the previous chapter and will now be considered in more detail. In a first study (Verhoef and Witter

1976), 40 µg of radioactively labelled Org 2766 was administered intravenously, subcutaneously, or orally. The uptake of radioactivity in the brain was very low for each of the three routes of administration (0.09–0.03 per cent of the dose/g brain tissue). The concentrations of intact peptide in the brain per gram fresh tissue were in the order of 10^{-4}–10^{-5} of the administered dose. Of course, it is possible that at specific sites much higher concentrations were present, as suggested in subsequent experiments, in which Org 2766 was injected intra-cerebroventricularly. This route of administration resulted in levels of intact peptide in the brain which were much higher than after systemic administration (at least 25 per cent of recovered radioactivity at two and four hours after injection) (Verhoef et al. 1977a). Further distribution studies were undertaken at two hours after intracerebroventricular injection. The septum accumulated most of the injected dose, followed in decreasing order by the hypothalamus and thalamus. This preferential uptake of the septum is in agreement with results from electrophysiological and lesion experiments. Urban (1977) elicited hippo-campal theta rhythm in rats by electrical stimulation of the reticular formation. Treatment with $ACTH_{4-10}$ accelerated theta activity, possibly due to increased excitability of the theta-generating reticuloseptohippocampal circuit. Also, lesions of the septum abolished the effect of $ACTH_{4-10}$ extinction (however, this was also true for lesions in some other brain structures, such as the hippocampus and the parafascicular nuclei of the thalamus) (Van Wimersma Greidanus 1977).

The possibility of transport from pituitary to the brain has been emphasized by results from an experiment in which radioactively-labelled Org 2766 was injected into the pituitary gland (Mezey et al. 1978). Radioactivity was recovered from many brain areas and transection of the pituitary stalk resulted in a decrease of uptake of Org 2766 into the brain; uptake was restored upon regeneration of the vascular connections. Thus, as suggested in the previous chapter, the vascular route seems to be important for carrying peptides from pituitary to brain. The cerebrospinal fluid may play a role too, for, when Org 2766 was injected into the space surrounding the pituitary gland, this was also followed by uptake of the peptide into the brain. Peptides can reach the median eminence from the pituitary through the vascular route, where they may enter the external fluid space, and from there the internal (cerebrospinal) fluid space. This route of transport may apply for peptides released from the pituitary, but also for peptides injected systemically, as the anterior pituitary is not covered by meninges (Palkovits and Mezey 1981).

Mechanism of action

The preferential uptake of Org 2766 into the septum is enhanced by hypo-physectomy (Verhoef et al. 1977b). $ACTH_{1-24}$ and $ACTH_{4-10}$, in contrast to α-endorphin and a vasopressin fragment, competed with the septal uptake of Org 2766. The investigators proposed that there are specific, high-affinity binding sites for ACTH-like peptides in the septum. However, so far these and possible other binding sites of ACTH in brain have not been identified and characterized. Watson and Akil (1981) reported that they have preliminary evidence that ACTH binds to brain with high affinity, although the number of binding sites is so low as to render a conclusive demonstration difficult (see also previous chapter).

Neurochemical investigations have suggested a number of neural processes with which ACTH-like peptides may interact, but none of these processes has been firmly linked yet to the behavioural effects of Org 2766. Information on the actions of ACTH-like peptides on brain amines is still fragmented and confusing. $ACTH_{1-10}$ and $ACTH_{4-10}$ have been found to increase noradrenalin and dopamine turnover in rat and mouse brain (Versteeg 1973; Leonard 1974; Dunn *et al.* 1976). At a less global level of analysis, ACTH-like peptides changed the functioning of dopamine neurons in two rat brain areas (Lichtensteiger and Monnet 1979). Functional alterations were assessed by microfluorimetry. The tuberoinfundibular neurons, which control MSH secretion, were influenced by α-MSH but not consistently by $ACTH_{4-10}$ or Org 2766. In contrast, intraperitoneal treatment with Org 2766 reduced the fluorescence of dopamine neurons in the substantia nigra; $ACTH_{4-10}$ and α-MSH were active to a lesser extent. The effect of Org 2766 was interpreted as a sign of decreased neuronal activity. The relevance of this finding for the behavioural activity of the peptide remains to be demonstrated.

It is commonly assumed that peptide hormones interact with receptors at the membranes of effector cells, thus enhancing intracellular levels of cyclic adenosine monophosphate (cAMP). The cyclic nucleotide, in turn, triggers a train of biochemical processes within the effector cell. There is some support for the view that changes in cAMP may mediate at least some of the behavioural actions of ACTH-like peptides. In a study by Wiegant and Gispen (1975), $ACTH_{1-10}$ increased cAMP levels in slices from rat posterior thalamus, including the parafascicular nuclei. This observation does not exclude the possibility that ACTH-like peptides may exert cAMP-independent effects. For example, it was shown that cAMP and $ACTH_{1-24}$ both altered *in vitro* phosphorylation of rat brain membrane proteins, but different protein bands were affected by these substances (Zwiers *et al.* 1976).

Changes in cAMP may alter brain macromolecular metabolism and, as described in the previous chapter, may provide another possible target for ACTH and related peptides. Hypophysectomized rats have deficient brain RNA and protein metabolism (Gispen and Schotman 1973), suggesting that hypophyseal peptides are involved in the regulation of brain macromolecule metabolism. The available data are consistent with an effect of behaviourally active ACTH-like peptides at the translational rather than the transcriptional level (cf. Gispen *et al.* 1977).

It should be noted that the effects described in this section concern acute treatment with Org 2766. The effects of chronic treatment may be different, as will be discussed in the next section.

Multiple effects of ACTH-like peptides

The behavioural effects discussed so far are shared by Org 2766, $ACTH_{4-10}$ and other ACTH-related peptides. There is evidence, however, that the profile of behavioural activity is not fully identical for all of these peptides. Some

ACTH-like peptides induce excessive grooming (scratching and licking of the fur), when injected intracerebroventricularly into rats (Wiegant *et al*. 1977) whilst some ACTH-like peptides have weak affinity to opiate receptors (Terenius *et al*. 1975). Org 2766 was inactive in these assays. The effects on grooming and on opiate receptors are therefore independent from the effects of these peptides on extinction, (passive) avoidance, and amnesia. This dissociation of behavioural profiles is illustrated by the Venn diagram in Fig. 8.5. Another example of dissociation, this syndrome of stretching and yawning, has been described in the previous chapter (Wood *et al*. 1978).

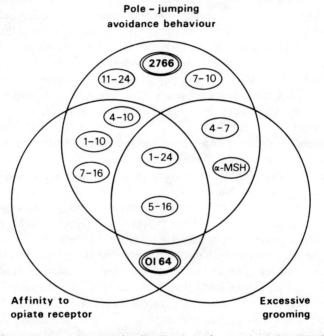

Fig. 8.5. Venn diagram showing the distribution of a number of ACTH-fragments and ACTH-analogues over three partially overlapping circles, representing three different biological activities. (Slightly modified from Greven and De Wied (1980), with kind permission.)

In the same manner as ACTH$_{4-10}$ and α-MSH (Fig. 8.5), Org 2766 may also exert multiple behavioural actions. This is suggested by the results of clinical studies with Org 2766 and studies with human volunteers (see previous chapter and Pigache and Rigter 1981). Acute administration of Org 2766 has been found to improve vigilance. This effect in man may well correspond with the effect of Org 2766, and other ACTH-like peptides, on attention/motivation in tests of extinction, amnesia, or passive avoidance in animals. Clinical data, however, suggest the existence of a second effect of Org 2766, which may or may not be related to the first one; this effect is only seen with chronic treatment, and is best described as an enhancement of mood. Almost all of the tests of Org 2766 and other ACTH-like peptides in animals have used acute administration of low doses of the peptide. Animal models for the mood-enhancing effect of Org 2766 probably should involve chronic treatment; these models have yet to be developed. An alternative strategy may be the use of acute but high doses of Org 2766. For instance, low and high doses of the peptide produced qualitatively different effects on retention of a passive avoidance response (Fekete and De Wied 1981).

In a recent animal study the chronic treatment regimen, as used in the clinic, was mimicked. The 2-deoxyglucose autoradiographic technique was employed to examine in rats the effects of chronic Org 2766 on local glucose utilization in the brain. Parts of the hippocampal formation, the anterior thalamus and anterior cingulate cortex, were identified as areas of possible functional involvement in the effects of Org 2766; In these structures increases in glucose utilization were observed (McCulloch *et al.* 1981). The number of areas influenced by the peptide was small, but they were all part of the limbic system. It may be that the effects of chronic Org 2766 are selective and specific and focused on the limbic system, notably the classical circuit of Papez.

Effects on mood

The available evidence suggests that the mood-enhancing effect of Org 2766 is not mediated through some action on opiate receptors. This is illustrated in Fig. 8.5. At first sight, the recent finding that microinjection of Org 2766 into the periaqueductal grey of rat brain produced analgesia (Walker *et al.* 1981), may be seen as support for an interaction of the peptide with opiate receptors. However, the opiate antagonist naloxone failed to reduce the analgesia and morphine tolerance did not diminish the effect of the peptide. In addition to this *in vivo* evidence for a non-opiate mechanism of action, Org 2766 even at high concentrations failed to inhibit the binding of [^{3}H]-naloxone to brain opiate receptors *in vitro*. Similarly, Org 2766 was ineffective at inhibiting [^{3}H]-β-endorphin binding to rat brain homogenates (Akil *et al.* 1980). Org 2766 also failed to affect brain opiate receptors when the peptide was chronically administered *in vivo*, by s.c. injection for 15 days. No substantial changes in binding of three ligands (dihydromorphine, [D-Ala, D-Leu] enkephalin, and etorphine) were found in eight brain areas (Messing, personal communication).

ORG 2766 AND AGING

The clinical data indicate that chronically administered Org 2766 is active in elderly subjects, although perhaps not exclusively so. It may be that aging produces (endocrine) deficits which can be corrected by peptide treatment. One possible deficit may concern the processing and production of behaviourally-active peptides, such as pro-OMC, described in the previous chapter. Pro-OMC is cleaved into fragments, many of which have behavioural activity. It is noteworthy that the fragment ACTH$_{4-10}$ is repeatedly present in the precursor molecule, as part of ACTH/α-MSH, γ-lipotropin and, slightly modified, in γ-MSH. The processing of the precursor molecule and its cleavage products may differ for different parts of the pituitary gland, or different parts of the brain (cf. Herbert *et al.* 1981).

The effects of aging on these recently discovered neuroendocrine processes remain to be established. There are data suggesting that in man hypothalamic-pituitary-adrenocortical function may be somewhat affected by aging, but not dramatically (cf. reviews by Blichert-Toft 1975; and Everitt 1980). Basal plasma glucocorticoid and ACTH levels are relatively normal in aged persons and the ACTH response to stress seems not to be compromised by age. Of course, it is possible that there are more subtle changes in hypothalamic–pituitary–adreno-cortical function which have gone largely undetected so far. Also, it is possible that the brain response to ACTH may change with aging, as suggested by results from experiments in rats (Landfield *et al.* 1980). Adrenalectomy reduced the occurrence of age-related neuroanatomical changes in the hippocampus, possibly through a feedback-dependent increase of ACTH. This possibility was substantiated by the finding that daily subcutaneous treatment with Org 2766 for a period of 9–10 months, also reduced hippocampal correlates of brain aging, in the absence of any alterations of steroids (Landfield *et al.* 1981).

There are a few indications that aging may alter processing of pro-OMC and its cleavage products. Thus, the amount of α-MSH in the hypothalamus of female rats has been found to decrease with age (Barnea *et al.* 1979). The β-endorphin content of all major rat brain areas known to contain this peptide, with the exception of the median eminence, was decreased approximately 50 per cent in old male rats compared to young rats (Barden *et al.* 1981). Hypothalamic levels of (Met) enkephalin were elevated in old male rats (Steger *et al.* 1980).

Acute and chronic effects

Further studies are needed to characterize the neuroendocrine changes that occur with aging, and to assess the relevance of such changes for the efficacy of Org 2766. The acute effect of the peptide in man, the increase in vigilance, has been assessed in young volunteers. The chronic, mood-enhancing effect of Org 2766 in man has been found in elderly subjects, although it may also occur in younger persons (see Pigache and Rigter 1981). Since it is probable that pharmacotherapy with Org 2766 will be indicated for elderly subjects more often than for young subjects, it is necessary to expand our knowledge about the effects of Org 2766 in aged organisms. At present, only two animal studies are available. In a first study (Rigter and Rijk, unpublished findings) a relatively high dose (2 mg/kg per day *per os*) of Org 2766 was given to male and female rats throughout their lives. The high dose was chosen, since the primary objective of the study was to determine whether Org 2766 had toxicological properties. No toxic effects of the peptide were detected. The continued dosing with Org 2766 did not affect life-span, and did not affect acquisition of maze and passive avoidance tasks at mid-life (14–16 months of age). When the animals had learned the maze problem (traversing the maze to obtain food), distracting stimuli were introduced (urine of unfamiliar rats not participating in the experiment). In the presence of distracting stimuli, Org 2766-treated male rats negotiated the maze with fewer errors than control animals, Thus, the peptide may have protected task performance against distraction. In addition, peptide treatment tended to improve retention of the maze task ($p < 0.1$), when retention was tested at 'old' age (nine months after acquisition, at 24 months of age). Org 2766 did not change behavioural performance of the female rats. This suggests a sex difference in rats in responsivity to the peptide.

A beneficial effect of chronic treatment with Org 2766 on performance of aged male rats on a maze task has also been reported by others (Landfield *et al.* 1981). These investigators confirmed that the peptide does not influence the learning of a maze problem. However, in their study, Org 2766 facilitated the subsequent learning of the mirror-image of the original maze problem (reversal test); the peptide corrected the deficit in reversal learning shown by the old rats. In yet another study (Rigter and Crabbe 1979), old male rats were again tested in the maze. The behaviour of the old rats during retention testing was different from that of young rats; the behavioural change could be reversed by an acute s.c. 0.1 µg/rat injection of Org 2766. This change was attributed to an exaggerated response to distracting stimuli irrelevant to the task.

The protection against distraction and the facilitation of reversal learning by Org 2766 may be just other examples of the influence of ACTH-like peptides on some process, or processes, akin to attention and motivation. The similar effects seen for both acute and chronic treatment testifies to this possibility. If so, this might mean that an animal correlate of the mood-enhancing effect of Org 2766 is yet to be demonstrated. Alternatively, it may be that the effects on attention/motivation and on mood are not basically different (for a discussion of the possible relationship between motivation and mood, see Pigache 1982).

CONCLUSIONS

Org 2766 is an analogue of ACTH$_{4-9}$, but it may be more than just a potent analogue; it may be a peptide with its own profile of behavioural activity. Org 2766 appears to exert two effects in man, an acute one on vigilance and a chronic one on mood. The acute effect on vigilance resembles many acute effects of Org 2766, shared by other ACTH-like peptides, in animals. These acute effects of the peptides in animals are commonly explained by a postulated change in attention or motivation. There is evidence that the reticulosepto-hippocampal circuit may be important for these acute effects. As yet, there is no convincing animal model for the mood-elevating effect of chronic treatment with Org 2766, although a few recent data offer promising perspectives. The mood-elevating effect of Org 2766 may be mediated through the classical circuit of Papez, comprising parts of the limbic system, and may be more pronounced in elderly than in young organisms. However, these hypotheses remain to be proven. At present, it is not clear if the acute and the chronic effects of Org 2766 are related.

REFERENCES

Akil, H., Hewlett, W. A., Barchas, J. D., and Li, C. C. (1980). Binding of ^{3}H-β-endorphin to rat brain membranes: characterization of opiate properties and interaction with ACTH. *Eur. J. Pharmac.* **64**, 1–8.

Barden, N., Dupont, A., Labrie, F., Mérand, Y., Rouleau, D., Vaudry, H., and Boissier, J. R. (1981). Age-dependent changes in the β-endorphin content of discrete rat brain nuclei. *Brain Res.* **208**, 209–12.

Barnea, A., Cho, G., and Porter, J. C. (1979). α-Melanocyte-stimulating hormone: a possible neuronal marker of the ageing brain. *J. Neurochem.* **33**, 1205–8.

Blichert-Toft, M. (1975). Secretion of corticotrophin and somatotrophin by the senescent adenohypophysis in man. *Acta endocr., Copenh.* Suppl., 195.

Bohus, B., Gispen, W. H., and De Wied, D. (1973). Effect of lysine vasopressin and ACTH$_{4-10}$ on conditioned avoidance behavior of hypophysectomized rats. *Neuroendocrinology* **11**, 137–43.

— Hendrickx, H. H. L., Van Kolfschoten, A. A., and Krediet, T. G. (1975). Effect of ACTH$_{4-10}$ on copulatory and sexually motivated approach behavior in the male rat. In *Sexual behavior: pharmacology and biochemistry* (ed. M. Sandler and G. L. Gessa) pp. 269–75. Raven Press, New York.

De Wied, D. (1969). Effects of peitide hormones on behavior. In *Frontiers in neuroendocrinology, 1969* (ed. W. F. Ganong and L. Martini) pp. 97–140. Oxford University Press, New York.

— (1977). Behavioral effects of neuropeptides related to ACTH, MSH and β-LPH. *Ann. NY Acad. Sci.* **297**, 263–74.

Dunn, A. J., Iuvone, P. M., and Rees, H. D. (1976). Neurochemical responses of mice to ACTH and lysine vasopressin. *Pharmac. Biochem. Behav.* **5** Suppl. 1, 139–45.

Everitt, A. V. (1980). The neuroendocrine system and aging. *Gerontology* **26**, 108–19.

Fekete, M. and De Wied, D. (1981). Effects of ACTH-4–10 and an ACTH-4–9 analogue (Org 2766) on avoidance behavior of rats. *Acta endocr., Copenh.* **97** Suppl. 243, no. 394.

Flood, J. F., Jarvik, M. E., Bennet, E. L., and Orme, A. E. (1976). Effects of ACTH peptide fragments on memory formation. *Pharmac. Biochem. Behav.* **5** Suppl. 1, 41–51.

Garrud, P., Gray, J. A., and De Wied, D. (1974). Pituitary–adrenal hormones and extinction of rewarded behaviour in the rat. *Physiol. Behav.* **12**, 109–19.

Gispen, W. H. and Schotman, P. (1973). Pituitary–adrenal system, learning and performance. Some neurochemical aspects. In *Drug effects on neuroendocrine regulation. Prog. Brain Res.* (ed. E. Zimmermann, W. H. Gispen, B. Marks, and D. De Wied) Vol. 39, pp. 443–9. Elsevier, Amsterdam.

— Van Ree, J. M., and De Wied, D. (1977). Lipotropin and the central nervous system. *Int. Rev. Neurobiol.* **20**, 209–50.

— Van Wimersma Greidanus, Tj. B., and De Wied, D. (1970). Effects of hypophysectomy and ACTH$_{1-10}$on responsiveness to electric shock in rats. *Physiol. Behav.* **5**, 143–7.

Gold, P. E. and McGaugh, J. L. (1977). Hormones and memory. In *Neuropeptide influences on the brain* (ed. L. H. Miller, C. A. Sandman, and A. J. Kastin) pp. 127–44. Raven Press, New York.

Greven, H. M. and De Wied, D. (1973). The influence of peptides derived from ACTH on performance. Structure activity studies. In *Drug effects on neuroendocrine regulation. Prog. Brain Res.* (ed. E. Zimmermann, W. H. Gispen, B. Marks, and D. De Wied) Vol. 39, pp. 443–59. Elsevier, Amsterdam.

— — (1980). Structure and behavioural activity of peptides related to corticotrophin and lipotrophin. In *Hormones and the brain* (ed. D. De Wied and P. A. Van Keep) pp. 115–26. MTP, Lancaster.

Herbert, E., Birnberg, N., Lissitsky, J.-C., Civelli, O., and Uhler, M. (1981). Pro-opiomelanocortin: a model for the regulation of expression of neuropeptides in pituitary and brain. *Neurosci. Comm.* **1**, 16–27.

Kastin, A. J., Dempsey, G. L., LeBlanc, B., Dyster-Aas, K., and Schally, A. V. (1974). Extinction of an appetitive operant response after administration of MSH. *Horm. Behav.* 5, 135-9.

Katz, R. J. (1980). Effects of an ACTH$_{4-9}$ related peptide upon intracranial self-stimulation and general activity in the rat. *Psychopharmacology* 71, 67-70.

Landfield, P. W., Baskin, R. K., and Pitler, T. A. (1981). Brain aging correlates: retardation by hormonal–pharmacological treatments. *Science, NY* 214, 581-4.

— Sundberg, D. K., Smith, M. S., Eldridge, J. C., and Movis, M. (1980). Mammalian aging: theoretical implications of changes in brain and endocrine systems during mid- and late-life in rats. *Peptides* 1 Suppl. 1, 185-96.

Leonard, B. E. (1974). The effect of two synthetic ACTH analogues on the metabolism of biogenic amines in the rat brain. *Archs Int. Pharmacodyn. Ther.* 207, 242-53.

Lichtensteiger, W. and Monnet, F. (1979). Differential response of dopamine neurons to α-melanotropin and analogues in relation to their endocrine and behavioral potency. *Life Sci.* 25, 2079-87.

Loeber, J. G., Van Wimersma Greidanus, Tj. B., and De Wied, D. (1979). Evidence for the existence of highly specific neuropeptides which affect the maintenance of avoidance behaviour. *J. Endocr.* 80, 9P.

McCulloch, J., Kelly, P. A. T., and Van Delft, A. M. L. (1981). The locus of action of a behaviorally active ACTH$_{4-9}$ analogue. *J. cereb. Blood Flow Metab.* 1 Suppl. 1, S490-1.

Mezey, E., Palkovits, M., De Kloet, E. R., Verhoef, J., and De Wied, D. (1978). Evidence for pituitary–brain transport of a behaviorally potent ACTH analog. *Life Sci.* 22, 831-8.

Palkovits, M. and Mezey, E. (1981). Anatomical connections between brain and anterior pituitary. In *ACTH and LPH in health and disease. Frontiers in hormone research* (ed. Tj. B. Van Wimersma Greidanus and L. H. Rees) Vol. 8, pp. 122-38. Karger, Basel.

Pigache, R. M. (1982). Effects of ACTH-like peptides on cognition and affect in the elderly. In *Neuropeptides and hormone modulation of brain function and homeostasis* (ed. J. M. Ordy, J. R. Sladek, and B. Reisberg). Raven Press, New York.

— and Rigter, H. (1981). Effects of peptides related to ACTH on mood and vigilance in man. In *Frontiers of hormone research. ACTH and LPH in health and disease* (ed. Tj. B. Van Wimersma Greidanus and L. H. Rees) Vol. 8, pp. 193-207. Karger, Basel.

Rigter, H. and Crabbe, J. C. (1979). Modulation of memory by pituitary hormones and related peptides. *Vitam. Horm.* 37, 153-241.

— Janssens-Elbertse, R., and Van Riezen, H. (1976). Reversal of amnesia by an orally active ACTH$_{4-9}$ analog (Org 2766). *Pharmac. Biochem. Behav.* 5 Suppl. 1, 53-8.

— and Popping, A. (1976). Hormonal influences on the extinction of conditioned taste aversion. *Psychopharmacologia* 46, 255-61.

— Van Riezen, H., and De Wied, D. (1974). The effects of ACTH- and vasopressin-analogues on CO_2-induced retrograde amnesia in rats. *Physiol. Behav.* 13, 381-8.

Sandman, C. A., Alexander, W. D., and Kastin, A. J. (1973). Neuroendocrine influences on visual discrimination and reversal learning in the albino and hooded rats. *Physiol. Behav.* 11, 613-17.

— and Kastin, A. J. (1977). Pituitary peptide influences on attention and memory. In *Neurobiology of sleep and memory* (ed. R. Drucker-Colin and J. L. McGaugh) pp. 347-60. Academic Press, New York.

Steger, R. W., Sonntag, W. E., Van Vugt, D. A., Forman, L. J., and Meites, J.

(1980). Reduced ability of naloxone to stimulate LH and testosterone release in aging male rats: possible relation to increase in hypothalamic met^5-enkephalin. *Life Sci.* **27**, 747–53.

Terenius, L., Gispen, W. H., and De Wied, D. (1975). ACTH-like peptides and opiate receptors in the rat brain: structure–activity studies. *Eur. J. Pharmac.* **33**, 395–9.

Urban, I. (1977). Electrophysiological correlates of behaviorally active neuropeptides: influence on hippocampal theta rhythm and paradoxical sleep. Ph. D. thesis, University of Utrecht.

Van Wimersma Greidanus, Tj. B. (1977). Effects of MSH and related peptides on avoidance behavior in rats. In *Frontiers of hormone research* (ed. Tj. B. Van Wimersma Greidanus) Vol. 4, pp. 129–39. Karger, Basel.

Verhoef, J., Palkovits, M., and Witter, A. (1977*a*). Distribution of a behaviorally highly potent ACTH$_{4-9}$ analog in rat brain after intraventricular administration. *Brain Res.* **126**, 89–104.

— and Witter, A. (1976). In vivo fate of a behaviorally active ACTH$_{4-9}$ analog in rats after systemic administration. *Pharmac. Biochem. Behav.* **4**, 583–90.

— — and De Wied, D. (1977*b*). Specific uptake of a behaviorally potent [^{3}H]-ACTH$_{4-9}$ analog in the septal area after intraventricular injection in rats. *Brain Res.* **131**, 117–28.

Versteeg, D. H. G. (1973). Effects of two ACTH-analogs on noradrenaline metabolism in rat brain. *Brain Res.* **49**, 483–5.

Walker, J. M., Berntson, G. G., Sandman, C. A., Kastin, A. J., and Akil, H. (1981). Induction of analgesia by central administration of Org 2766, an analog of ACTH$_{4-9}$. *Eur. J. Pharmac.* **69**, 71–9.

Watson, S. J. and Akil, H. (1981). Anatomical and functional studies of ACTH and lipotropin in central nervous system. In *ACTH and LPH in health and disease. Frontiers of hormone research* (ed. Tj. B. Van Wimersma Greidanus and L. H. Rees) Vol. 8, pp. 149–61. Karger, Basel.

Wiegant, V. M. and Gispen, W. H. (1975). Behaviourally active ACTH-analogues and brain cyclic AMP. *Exp. Brain Res.* **23** Suppl., 219.

— — Terenius, L., and De Wied, D. (1977). ACTH-like peptides and morphine interaction at the level of the CNS. *Psychoneuroendocrinology* **2**, 63.

Witter, A., Greven, H. M., and De Wied, D. (1975). Correlation between structure, behavioral activity and rate of biotransformation of some ACTH$_{4-9}$ analogs. *J. Pharmac. exp. Ther.* **193**, 853–60.

Wood, P. L., Malthe-Sørenssen, D., Cheney, D. L., and Costa, E. (1978). Increase of hippocampal acetylcholine turnover rate and the stretching–yawning syndrome elicited by alpha-MSH and ACTH. *Life Sci.* **22**, 673–8.

Zwiers, H., Veldhuis, H. D., Schotman, P., and Gispen, W. H. (1976). ACTH, cyclic nucleotides, and brain protein phosphorylation in vitro. *Neurochem. Res.* **1**, 669–77.

9

Drug treatment of senile dementia

RICHARD J. McDONALD

INTRODUCTION

A variety of psychopharmacological drugs are prescribed for the treatment of cognitive, behavioural, and emotional symptoms which are thought to accompany senile dementia. Even though the aetiology of this disease is not well understood, it is generally presumed to be caused by neurophysiological changes in the brain. Therefore a psychopharmacological approach is taken. The intention and hope of this endeavour is that the drugs may ameliorate or even reverse the disabilities of this tragic state.

The psychopharmacological treatment of these disorders usually involves the administration of either one of the major classes of psychotropic agents or gerontopsychopharmacological agents. Loew and Vigouret report that the latter drugs in contrast with the classic psychotropic drugs, have 'specific effects on the central nervous system that suggest they would be of particular value in the treatment of behavioural and mental disturbances often occurring in old people' (1981). Reviews addressing the effectiveness of psychotropic agents have been covered extensively (Ban 1980; Hicks *et al.* 1980; Reisberg *et al.* 1980; Wittenborn 1981) and are not dealt with in this article. Rather, the focus of the chapter will be an in-depth review of two gerontopsychopharmacological agents: co-dergocrine mesylate (hydergine) and piracetam, and an assessment of their relative clinical merits.

Before reviewing a large number of pharmacological attempts designed with the hope of alleviating or inhibiting the symptoms of senile dementia, a few comments regarding the current methods used in the assessment and evaluation of the efficacy of treatment of these disorders are warranted. It should be kept in mind that there is no perfect methodology for the clinical evaluation of drug treatment in the elderly, and the techniques employed have advantages as well as limitations. Therefore, when examining results of the drug studies presented, it is necessary to do so in light of the methodology that was applied. Familiarity with the various research tools utilized, and awareness of their strengths and weaknesses, should afford the clinician a better understanding of the results presented and their applications.

MEASURING DRUG EFFECTS

Clinical rating scales

Clinical rating scales are the principal instruments used in geriatric psychopharmacological research (Venn 1978). In comprehensive reviews by Salzman *et al.*

(1972) and updated by Honigfeld (1982), it was reported that there are 39 scales suitable for evaluation of geriatric patients and 17 are designed specifically for geriatric psychiatric populations. Although a few of these instruments have been used in geriatric psychopharmacological investigations, it is noteworthy that only one of the scales (Sandoz Clinical Assessment Geriatric scale (SCAG); Shader *et al.* 1974), was specifically designed for this type of research with the elderly (Kochansky 1979; Venn 1978). Before describing the SCAG it may be worthwhile to comment on the advantages and limitations of observer-rating instruments.

The advantages of observer-rating techniques used in an interview situation, are that clinicians are free to assess the status of the patient from a range of behavioural and affective cues, both verbal and non-verbal. Likewise, they are in a position to direct the flow of events and, when necessary, they are able to gain additional clarification of responses, behaviours, and feelings. Also, since raters (it is assumed) are clinically well-trained individuals, they are able to elicit more information and detect subtle changes. In addition, the validity of the observations may be increased due to the clinician–patient proximity and the immediacy of the rating (Derogatis *et al.* 1972; Honigfeld 1982).

Limitations of such techniques are that a clinician's sphere of reference is usually limited to the immediate situation. This may in turn restrict the rater's perception and thus the evaluation may not be an accurate reflection of the patient's total behaviour. Likewise, in interview situations it is possible that episodic behaviour will not be evaluated, and also there is no direct observation of social behaviour and performance of daily activities. In addition, the co-operation of the patient is required (Derogatis *et al.* 1972; Gottschalk 1975; Honigfeld 1982).

Other factors suggestive of decreasing the reliability and validity of these techniques are various measurement problems, e.g., halo effects, error of central tendency, leniency error (Anastasi 1976; Wittenborn 1967, 1972). A final measurement problem concerns the subjective elements involved in assessing behaviour in an interview situation via rating scales. It is reported that clinicians' judgments are influenced by their theoretical orientation, age, school of thought, and personality (Katz *et al.* 1969; Yager 1977; Gauron and Dickinson 1969). Even more prevalent are the expectations that clinicians may have about elderly people and their capacities (Bulter 1975; Bulter and Lewis 1977; Karasu *et al.* 1979; Shader *et al.* 1979). The elderly are often depicted as suffering from severe organic defects and depressive disorders. Such expectations may have a negative influence on clinicians' ratings and therefore decrease the reliability of these assessments. Being cognizant of important characteristics of the elderly, coupled with good interviewing techniques, should reduce variability and enhance the clinician's ability to evaluate the effects of treatment. Suggestions for practising interviewing skills are provided by Gurland (1980).

The Sandoz Clinical Assessment Geriatric scale

The SCAG, an observer-rating instrument, is the only standard multiple psycho- pathological rating scale designed specifically for geriatric patients (Kochansky 1979). It was developed by Sandoz Pharmaceuticals in order to provide a standard

TABLE 9.1. *Sandoz Clinical Assessment Geriatric Scale (SCAG)**

1. Confusion	11. Bothersome
2. Mental alertness	12. Indifference to surroundings
3. Impairment of recent memory	13. Unsociability
4. Orientation	14. Unco-operativeness
5. Mood depression	15. Fatigue
6. Emotional lability	16. Appetite
7. Self-care	17. Dizziness
8. Motivation–initiative	18. Anxiety
9. Irritability	19. Overall impression of patient
10. Hostility	

*From Shader *et al.* (1974).

reliable, easy-to-use, general-purpose rating scale for evaluating the efficacy of drug treatment (Venn 1978). The SCAG consists of 18 symptoms (Table 9.1) and an overall impression area, all rated on a seven-point format (1 = not present; 4 = mild to moderate; 7 = severe) (Shader *et al.* 1974, p. 107; Venn 1978, pp. 540-1). Raters are instructed on the manner in which the symptoms should be evaluated, by way of a short description of each item and whether the item is rated on the patient's responses and statements at the interview, or on observed behaviour at and/or outside the interview.

A few factor-analytic studies of the SCAG have been undertaken (Gaitz *et al.* 1977; Shader *et al.* 1979; Singer and Hamot 1980) with the latter being the most comprehensive one. It was based upon the pretreatment SCAG scores for 1109 patients. The factor analysis yielded six factors and explained about 65 per cent of the variance. In the study by Gaitz *et al.* (1977), a principal axis factor analysis was computed for all subjects (*N*:47) across all time periods (pretreatment 3, 6, 9, 12, 15, 18, 21, and 24 weeks). This analysis resulted in four factors. Shader *et al.* (1979) in their factor analytic methods, based on scores for 37 ambulatory volunteers, identified five factors which accounted for 63 per cent of the total SCAG variance. The findings for these three factor analytic studies are presented in Table 9.2.

As shown in Table 9.2, the factor content of the Singer and Hamot study is comparable to that reported earlier by Gaitz *et al.*, noting, however, they labelled two factors differently, i.e. interpersonal relationship = agitation/irritability, and apathy = withdrawal. The major difference was that Gaitz *et al.* found a factor of *mood depression* whereas Singer and Hamot clustered these items into the factors *affective* and *somatic functioning.* The cluster analysis of Shader *et al.* differed somwhat from the other two. It is worth keeping in mind that the above three factor analyses are based on different sample populations and that this may have, in part, accounted for the different structures.

In spite of these differences, it is apparent that the SCAG may be organized into different factors thus allowing for more understanding of treatment efficacy. Gaitz *et al.* (1977) demonstrated this by showing that positive changes in cognitive function, cannot be accounted for as a mere reflection of improved mood and general well-being. Likewise, Singer and Hamot (1980) have demonstrated

TABLE 9.2. *Summary of the factor analytic studies of the Sandoz Clinical Assessment Geriatric scale (SCAG)*

A. SCAG factor structure according to Singer and Hamot (1980)

Interpersonal relationships	Cognitive dysfunction	Affective	Apathy	Somatic functioning	Self-care
Co-operation	Mental alertness	Emotional lability	Motivation/initiative	Appetite	Self-care
Irritability	Confusion	Depression	Indifference to surroundings	Dizziness	
Bothersome	Recent memory	Anxiety	Unsociability	Fatigue	
Hostility	Orientation				

B. SCAG factor scores according to Gaitz et al. (1977)

Agitation/irritability	Cognitive dysfunction	Mood depression	Withdrawal
Emotional lability	Confusion	Mood depression	Motivation/initiative
Irritability	Mental alertness	Fatigue	Indifference to surroundings
Hostility	Recent memory	Appetite	Unsociability
Bothersomeness	Disorientation	Dizziness	
Unco-operativeness	Self-care	Anxiety	

C. SCAG five clusters according to Shader et al. (1979)

Confusion	Memory impairment	Indifference	Bothersomeness	Mood
Confusion	Impairment of recent memory	Disorientation	Bothersomeness	Anxiety
Mental alertness	Fatigue	Motivation/initiative	Unco-operativeness	Mood depression
	Dizziness	Indifference to surroundings	Appetite	Emotional lability
		Self-care		Irritability
				Hostility
				Unsociability

the usefulness of applying cluster analysis of the SCAG in discriminating between senile dementia and depression in groups of elderly patients. Concern, however, has been voiced about the SCAG because of two omissions: 'There is no standard administration instruction to assure at least a systematic interview period, and there are no guidelines presented to provide a consistent frame of reference' (Shader *et al.* 1979, p. 155). Similar points were raised by McDonald (1979) in an earlier review of hydergine studies. Also of interest would be information regarding the sensitivity of the scale in rating ambulatory samples, the stability of ratings over time, normative data for different diagnostic groups, and the relationship of the ratings with psychometric parameters and physiological measurements. Such information would add further support to the usefulness of this instrument in evaluating drug or other treatment effects in elderly patients.

Psychometry

Psychometric tests are designed to provide a descriptive pattern of an individual's strengths and weaknesses of specific functions (Kramer and Jarvik 1979). Since they are more directly related to cerebral function, they offer a more objective assessment of behavioural and cognitive functions than, for example, rating scales. There is a multiplicity of psychometric tests available, measuring numerous aspects of cerebral functions, ranging from elementary ones to complex activities. Common tests performed are: simple and complex reaction time tests, psychomotor tests, auditory and visual perception tests, continuous performance tests, intelligence tests, memory and cognitive function tests. Such tests may be given individually, or a more popular approach has been to select a battery of tests. By administering two or more tests, one is not only able to observe performance on a number of tests, but more importantly, one has a basis to compare relationships, trends, and discrepancies among the tests (for reviews see Kramer and Jarvik 1979; Miller 1980, 1981; Wells and Buchanan 1979).

In the last few years there has been an increase in the use of psychometric tests in geriatric psychopharmacological research. Examples of assembled test batteries are provided by Lloyd-Evans *et al.* (1978). McConnachie (1978), and Oswald (1979). Additional test batteries are the Wechsler Adult Intelligence Scale (WAIS; Wechsler 1955), the Short WAIS (Savage *et al.* 1973), and the Wechsler Memory Scale (Wechsler 1945). The following section highlights a number of test batteries which are being used in geriatric psychopharmacological research.

The WAIS is one of the most widely used clinical tests, is age-adjusted, and has proven useful in the assessment of dementia. The WAIS is made up of 11 subtests, six verbal: information, arithmetic, similarities, comprehension, digit span, vocabulary; and five performance: digit symbol, picture completion, block design, picture arrangement, object assembly. Performances on both the verbal and performance subtests are combined to form respective scores, and a full score is the combination of the two. A deterioration index may also be computed.

The Wechsler Memory Scale (WMS) assesses a wide span of memory functions. It consists of seven subtests: personal and current information, orientation, mental control, logical memory, digit span, visual reproduction, and associate learning. The test is designed to determine a memory quotient. It is widely used, but Kramer and Jarvik (1979) as well as Wells and Buchanan (1979) concluded that its use far exceeds its usefulness. A few drug studies have employed this index (Crook *et al.* 1977; Ferris *et al.* 1977; Westreich *et al.* 1975), but reported no changes on WMS performance due to drug therapy.

The Nuremberg Geriatric Inventory (NGI; Oswald 1979) is a battery of tests designed to measure various behavioural aspects of the elderly, e.g. test performance, mood, daily activities, and attitudes. It is intended for use in geriatric psychopharmacological research. The test is comprised of three modified subtests of the WAIS: digit span, block design, and digit-symbol test; a maze test, a recognition test, a modified trail-making test, a rating scale for activities of daily living, and various self-rating scales assessing attitudes, state of being, and a comparison of today's status with that of last year. The inventory or segments of it have been administered in pharmacological investigations (Kugler *et al.* 1978; Oswald and Lang 1980).

The Mental Status Check List (MSCL; Lifschitz 1960) is an easily administered test designed to measure intellectual abilities and mental acuity. The test consists of 17 questions which measure the subject's ability to do successive subtractions, give general information, identify objects, comprehend abstraction, and write a sentence. The test may be administered in either a standardized testing situation or the information may be elicited during an informal conversation.

Branconnier and Cole (1978) derived an overall impairment index from a battery of 10 neuropsychological tests and a self-rating adjective checklist. Tests employed were spatial orientation, concept formation, motor performance, memory, visual perception, and mood. Scores obtained were normalized, converted to probits, and summed to yield an impairment index. The authors claim it is reasonable to employ a symptom-independent index to assess drug efficacy in senile dementia, because patients vary in both type and intensity, therefore the single index is a sensitive indicator of the amelioration of symptoms.

Psychometric tests are indicators of important cerebral functions and should be acknowledged as a potential assessment method of treatment-related changes. It is worth noting, however, that many variables may intervene to influence the performance of the aged on these tests, and thus limit their usefulness. Prominent ones cited, are the patient's motivation and willingness to perform (Botwinick 1973; Welford 1976), their perception of the task relevancy (Botwinick 1973), their anxiety-arousal level (Eisdorfer 1968; Schaie 1968), their perceived health status (Kahn *et al.* 1975; McDonald and Suchy 1980), their disease state (Lezak 1976; Yesavage *et al.* 1979b), sensory and motor changes occurring with advanced age (Corso 1977; Fozard *et al.* 1977; Welford 1977, 1980). There are also situational variables in test-taking, such as fatigue-producing conditions (Fury and Baltes 1973), and irrelevant stimuli (Rabbit 1965). In addition, other methodological issues are present, i.e. the validity of the tests, namely construct, criterion-related, and contextual validity (Crook 1979).

It is evident that motivational, sensory, affective, and disease factors significantly influence the psychometric performance of the elderly and affect an instrument's capacity to reflect the component or constructs it intends to measure. Therefore, in order to enhance the usefulness of psychometric tests it is necessary to acquire familiarity with the various tests and an appreciation of the many factors that produce deviations in performance.

Physiological measurement

The electroencephalogram (EEG) is an important non-invasive diagnostic procedure in evaluating age-related disorders. Its sensitivity to brain functions makes it a valuable diagnostic tool in assessing patients with confusion, dementia, and depression (Wilson *et al.* 1977). Likewise, it is becoming a valuable tool in demonstrating and characterizing the therapeutic effects of pharmacological agents (Matejcek 1980). This, coupled with the development of more sophisticated computer-aided techniques, has opened up a new promising field of research in brain activity. An example is reported by Matejcek (1980). The EEGs of 619 subjects aged 45–95 years were evaluated by spectral analysis (three-minute resting EEG, lead O_2-C_2). The EEG analysis identified a significant age-related increase in slow frequencies, namely those in the delta and theta bands and a significant decrease in alpha and beta activity. These EEG changes helped to formulate a working hypothesis that 'centrally acting drugs with the ability to counteract age-related EEG changes might bring about a clinically relevant improvement in the symptoms associated with functional deterioration of the CNS' (Matejcek 1980, p. 342). The results of studies designed to test this hypothesis (Kugler *et al.* 1978; Matejcek *et al.* 1979) are presented in the next section.

Radioisotope techniques are another physiological method employed in this field in order to monitor changes in the cerebral circulation time and to observe changes in transit time after treatment. They are safe and reliable methods for repeated measures of the cerebral-blood perfusion rate (Mongeau 1974).

HYDERGINE

Hydergine is a preparation containing equal parts of the mesylates of the ergot derivatives dihydroergocorine, dihydroergocristine, and dihydroergokryptine (Fig. 9.1). It has been marketed since the early fifties by Sandoz Pharmaceuticals, and is probably the best studied, reviewed, and one of the most widely prescribed preparations for the treatment of elderly patients. A recent survey by Zawadski *et al.* (1978) reported that among Medicaid aged in California, hydergine was second to thioridazine in terms of drug expenditures among the institutionalized population. At present it is the only drug fully approved by the Food and Drug Administration for clinical use in treatment of idiopathic mental disorders of aging (FDC Reports 1979).

Hydergine was initially thought to be, and developed as, a peripheral vasodilator (Venn 1978); but it is now thought to benefit brain cell metabolism and brain synaptic transmission (Loew 1980). Reisberg (1981) classifies hydergine as a cerebral metabolic enhancer. The pharmacological effects of hydergine have been extensively studied and succinctly summarized by Loew (1980). It is reported that hydergine increases the activity of certain enzymes of intermediary metabolism in ganglion cells, alters glucose stores in astrocytes,

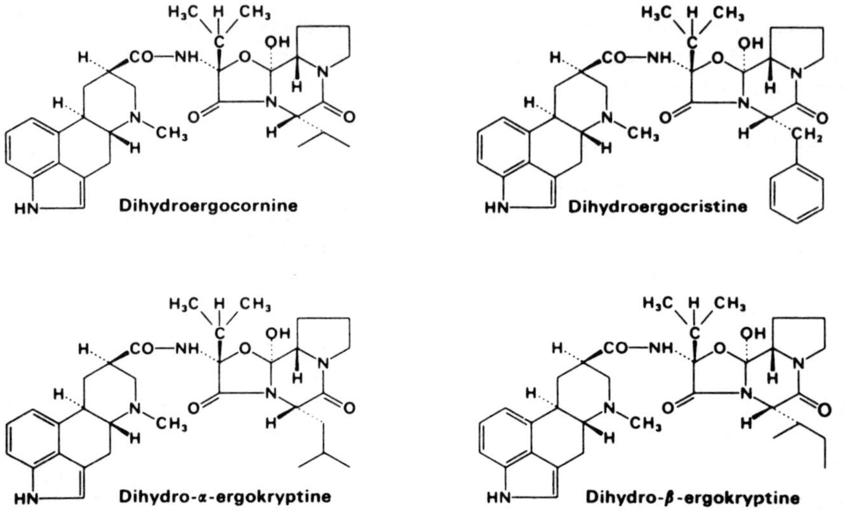

Fig. 9.1. Chemical structure of the four dihydrogenated ergot peptide derivatives which, in their methanesulphonate (mesylate) form, constitute dihydroergotoxine mesylate.

increases cerebral oxygen utilization, and increases EEG amplitudes (Meier-Ruge *et al.* 1975). In addition, in acute animal experiments there is no clear-cut evidence that hydergine increases cerebral blood-flow (CBF), but in cats with reduced CBF it augments electrical power of the electrocortigram (Meier-Ruge *et al.* 1978). Recent work on brain monoamine receptors, indicates it binds to rat brain receptor sites specific for noradrenalin, dopamine, and serotonin (Loew *et al.* 1979). Hydergine also counteracts noradrenalin-induced cyclic AMP elevations in the rat brain cortex (Markstein and Wagner 1978) and has dopamine agonist effects (Loew *et al.* 1979). The rationale for its clinical use is that some patients with senile dementia have a defect in neuronal intermediary metabolism. By ameliorating this fault, it is speculated that mentation, EEG activity, and cerebral blood-flow would also improve (Yesavage *et al.* 1979*b*, p. 221).

Methdology of studies

Table 9.3 presents an overview of methodological characteristics employed in the hydergine studies, and lists the number of variables which showed a significant improvement ($p \leqslant 0.05$) in the hydergine group, in comparison with the control group. All studies included in this review appeared in the public domain after 1968.

All investigations were conducted under double-blind (DB) conditions and two of them (Biel *et al.* 1976; Rehman 1973) utilized a cross-over design. As shown in the table, placebo was the comparison substance used most often (N:27). Five trialists elected to compare hydergine with papaverine, two compared hydergine plus acetyldigoxin with acetyldigoxin alone, and the others compared it with either piribedil, chlordiazepoxide, or multivitamins. Yesavage *et al.* (1981) opted to examine the treatment of senile dementia with hydergine combined with either supportive counselling or cognitive training

Most of the samples were selected on the criteria that the patients concerned were manifesting a mild to moderate degree of symptoms, attributed to or associated with either cerebral arteriosclerosis, cerebrovascular insufficiency, senile mental deterioration, or dementia. Clinical symptoms describing these diagnostic indications were usually categorized under the headings: impairment of cognitive functions, dysphoric mood states, and impairment of behavioural functioning. Excluded were patients with psychosis, post-traumatic brain damage, postinfective brain disease, cerebral neoplasm, or other conditions which might interfere with the clinical assessment.

In total, 1,979 patients were included in the 38 DB studies, and 52 per cent received hydergine. Slightly more than 60 per cent of the patients were females (based upon sex distribution data presented in 30 studies), the mean ages of the samples ranged from 63 to 85 years and, pooled together it was 76 years. Patients were either residing in hospitals (42 per cent), nursing homes/old age homes (39 per cent), or were outpatients (19 per cent). The daily dosage for 25 studies was 3 mg and for 13 studies 4.5 mg. Medication was administered either as sublingual tablets, tablets, or drops before, during, or after meals. The duration for 25 studies was 12 weeks, whereas for nine studies the evaluation period varied from four to eight weeks. The remaining four studies extended for a longer time period, ranging from six months up to a maximum of 15 months. Appraisals in these studies were usually made at monthly or bimonthly intervals.

Various statistical procedures were computed on the data collected in these studies. The results presented in this review are based primarily upon the significant differences between treatment groups as determined by analysis of variance or analysis of covariance. The main assessment methods employed were either clinical rating scales, psychometric tests, physiological measurements, or a combination of two or more of these research instruments. Clinical rating scales were by far the primary tool chosen to evaluate the efficacy of hydergine. Every investigator, except for two (Kugler *et al.* 1978; Oswald and Lang 1980), used some type of clinical rating scale. The SCAG or an earlier version of it was utilized in 24 investigations. Apart from the SCAG, the Crichton Royal Behavioural Rating Scale and other ward behavioural rating scales, i.e. general-purpose scales assessing social competence and daily living activities, were used in these trials. Psychometric testing consisted of the Mental Status Check List which was administered in 12 studies. Other tests performed were subtests of the WAIS, e.g. digit span, digit symbol, and other performance tests, both power and speed ones. Physiological measurements were radioisotope techniques and the EEG. The EEG was recorded in seven studies and cerebral circulation time was measured in two studies.

Results with hydergine

As shown in Table 9.3 almost all of the studies reported varying degrees of success with hydergine therapy over the comparison substance, as determined by clinical rating scales. In 19 of the 36 studies at least half of the tested symptoms or symptom clusters, showed significant hydergine–control differences.

TABLE 9.3. *Summary of the hydergine studies, N = 38*

Author(s)	Year	Setting	N	x̄ age	Hydergine daily doses	Comparison substance	Duration (weeks)	Results* Rating scale	Psychometry	Physiology	Global rating
Arrigo et al.	1973	Hospital	20	68	4.5 mg	Placebo	12	5/18	–	EEG–NS	S
Banen	1972	Hospital	77	–	3.0 mg	Placebo	12	3/20	0/5	–	NS
Bargheon	1973	–	109	74	4.5 mg	Placebo	12	13/17	–	–	–
Bazo	1973	Nursing home	66	85	3.0 mg	Papaverine†	12	4/17	2/7	–	NS
Biel et al.	1976	Old age home	51	79	3.0 mg	Placebo	6+6	3/7	–	EEG–S	–
Bochner et al.	1973	Hospital	21	64	3.0 mg	Placebo	12	0/21	0/7	–	S
Chudnovsky	1979	Outpatients	72	70	3.0 mg	Placebo	24	6/18	–	–	S
Cox et al.	1978	Hospital	28	–	4.5 mg	Placebo	12	S	S	–	S
Dennler and Bachmann	1979	–	80	63	3.0 mg‡	Acetyldigoxin	8	3/6	–	–	S
Ditch et al.	1971	Hospital	39	85	3.0 mg	Placebo	12	2/30	–	–	NS
Einspruch	1976	Nursing home	39	81	3.0 mg	Papaverine†	12	6/18	–	–	NS
Gaitz et al.	1977	Nursing home	47	–	3.0 mg	Placebo	24	11/18	0/6	–	S
Gerin	1969	Old age home	39	82	3.0 mg	Placebo	12	S	NS	–	–
Grill and Broicher	1969	Hospital	54	70	3.0 mg	Placebo	6	9/11	–	–	–
Heiss et al.	1969	Outpatients	60	65	3–4.5 mg	Placebo	12	5/20	4/20	–	S
Herzfeld et al.	1972	Hospital	55	–	3–4.5 mg	Placebo	6	10/17	4/9	EEG, CBF	–
Hollingsworth	1980	Nursing home	53	79	3.0 mg	Placebo	12	10/18	0/6	–	NS
Jennings	1972	Hospital	50	80	3.0 mg	Placebo	12	8/17	0/6	–	S
Kugler et al.	1978	Old age home	100	77	4.5 mg	Placebo	60	–	2/9	EEG, CBF	–
Linden	1975	Outpatients	50	78	3.0 mg	Placebo	12	17/18	0/6	–	S
Matejcek et al.	1979	Hospital	16	76	4.5 mg	Placebo	12	2/18	–	EEG–S	NS

	Year	Setting			Dose	Comparison	n				Result*
McConnachie	1973	Old age home	52	81	4.5 mg	Placebo	12	S	–	–	S
Nelson	1975	In-/outpatients	45	78	3.0 mg	Papaverine†	12	12/16	0/6	–	S
Nicrosini and Pasotti	1976	–	60	75	4.5 mg	Piribedil	4	0/21	0/6	–	–
Oswald and Lang	1980	Old age home	34	74	3.0 mg	Chlordiazepoxide	6	–	2/3	–	–
Pfeiff et al.	1980	Old age home	87	80	3.0 mg‡	Acetyldigoxin	8	3/13	5/7	–	NS
Rao and Norris	1972	Hospital	57	78	3.0 mg	Placebo	12	12/18	2/6	–	S
Rehmann	1973	Hospital	46	83	4.5 mg	Placebo	8/8	0/10	–	–	NS
Rehmann	1973	Hospital	30	78	4.5 mg	Placebo	12	4/10	–	–	S
Rosen	1975	Outpatients	53	66	3.0 mg	Papaverine†	12	13/15	0/6	–	S
Roubicek et al.	1972	Hospital	44	79	4.5 mg	Placebo	12	9/18	S	EEG–S	S
Short and Benway	1972	Hospital	49	83	3.0 mg	Placebo	12	10/17	0/6	–	S
Soni and Soni	1975	Outpatients	78	69	4.5 mg	Multivitam.	36	S	–	–	–
Thibault	1974	Nursing home	48	80	3.0 mg	Placebo	12	13/18	–	–	–
Triboletti and Ferri	1969	Nursing home	59	79	3.0 mg	Placebo	12	5/25	0/6	–	–
Wilder and Gonyea	1973	Hospital	28	68	3.0 mg	Placebo	6	6/17	–	EEG–S	S
Winslow	1974	Hospital	53	79	3.0 mg	Papaverine†	12	17/18	3/7	–	S
Yesavage et al.§	1981	Outpatients	20	68	3.0 mg	Hydergine	12	11/18	S	–	S

*Results: number of variables which showed a significant improvement, $p \leq 0.05$, in the Hydergine group in comparison with the other treatment group.

†Papaverine: daily dose 300 mg.

‡Hydergine: Hydergine plus 1 mg Acetyldigoxin.

§Yesavage et al.: Treatment groups – Hydergine plus cognitive training or Hydergine plus supportive counselling.

In 18 of the 26 studies appraising global change, significant improvement with hydergine was demonstrated. On the other hand, three studies (Bochner *et al.* 1973; Nicrosini and Pasotti 1976; Rehmann 1973) reported no significant between-group differences, and an additional three (Banen 1972; Ditch *et al.* 1971; Matejcek *et al.* 1979) indicated that less than one-sixth of the rating scale items reached a $p \le 0.05$ level of significance.

Table 9.4 summarizes the significant results obtained with the SCAG or close modifications of it. The factor structure of the SCAG is according to Singer and Hamot (1980). Using the criterion that a symptom shows significant improvement in 50 per cent of the studies in which it was tested, 13 of the 18 SCAG symptoms improved significantly with hydergine. All symptoms clustered in the factor headings 'cognitive dysfunction' and 'affective', showed positive improvement in at least 50 per cent of the studies. The symptoms 'depression, confusion, and disorientation' were the ones which had the highest proportion of improvement. Hughes *et al* (1976) found in their review of 12 studies, a significant improvement in 10 of the 18 symptoms, and based upon a review of 26 studies, McDonald (1979) reported that 11 symptoms reached this level.

TABLE 9.4. *Summary of the SCAG results and the fraction of studies reporting a significant (*p $\le$ 0.05*) improvement with Hydergine in comparison with other treatment group. The denominator indicates the number of studies which specifically stated the symptom was assessed as an individual item*

Cognitive dysfunction			**Affective**	
Mental alertness	8/16		Emotional lability	13/22
Confusion	12/18		Depression	19/27
Recent memory	10/16		Anxiety	10/15
Disorientation	10/15			
			Apathy	
Interpersonal relationships			Motivation/initiative	11/20
Co-operation	9/23		Indifference to surroundings	4/15
Irritability	9/18		Unsociability	12/21
Bothersome	7/14			
Hostility	7/16		**Somatic functioning**	
			Appetite	8/22
Self-care			Dizziness	13/24
Self-care	9/23		Fatigue	12/23

Factor structure of the SCAG based upon the factor analysis of 1109 patients: pretreatment scores. (From Singer and Hamot (1980).)

The findings of the mental status check list (Table 9.5) were in sharp contrast with the clinical rating scale findings. In 12 studies, this performance test was administered and seldom were significant group differences obtained, on any of the mental abilities tapped by this objective test instrument. Positive changes, however, were observed on other psychometric tests in the hydergine-treated groups. In particular, performance improved on some of the WAIS subtests, e.g. digit span, and Kugler *et al.* (1978) reported a significant difference in the WAIS total score following 15 months of hydergine therapy. There were also

TABLE 9.5. *Summary of the psychometry and physiological findings*

Mental status checklist	
Orientation	2/12
Successive subtractions	1/12
General information	0/12
Object information	1/12
Abstraction	2/12
Writing performance	0/12
EEG – increase in alpha frequency decrease in slow activity	
CBF – decrease in total time	

slight indications that hydergine favourably improved performance on certain speed tests.

EEG changes reported in seven studies were in agreement with one another and in five of these studies significant differences were found. Similarities registered in the EEG recordings were an increase in alpha activity, 8–10 Hz, and a decrease in the theta and delta ranges. Matejcek *et al.* (1979) also found a reduction in the relative power of the beta frequencies, but the power in the delta and theta ranges did not vary significantly. Regarding CBF, both investigators reported improvement, i.e. cerebral circulation time was shortened and stabilized. Side-effects or significant changes in vital signs were seldom reported. All investigators unanimously concluded hydergine to be a safe and well-tolerated drug.

Interpretation of the findings

In summary it appears that hydergine is influential in alleviating or inhibiting certain target symptoms associated with senile dementia, as detected by clinicians using behavioural rating scales. In particular, the compilation of the data reveals, in the statistical sense, that improvement is mainly in the areas of cognitive dysfunction and mood depression. Unclear is the mechanism of action. For example, does hydergine act primarily as an antidepressant, thus improving mood, with positive changes in cognitive functions being only secondary? Also, does hydergine provide long-term benefit in the treatment of these disorders and is there an optimal dosage? An attempt will be made to provide clarification regarding these issues.

The first point regarding the therapeutics of hydergine has generated much speculation and controversy. Work conducted by Shader and co-workers (Shader and Goldsmith 1976; Shader *et al.* 1979) supports the possibility that antidepressant activity may be a contributing factor in the efficacy of hydergine. They compared hydergine (3 mg, N:9) to imipramine (75–100 mg, N:13), and placebo (N:14), in ambulatory geriatric patients with a mild degree of mood and cognitive impairment. The results with both drugs did not vary from placebo for seven weeks, but were both significant after nine weeks of therapy (Fig. 9.2). No evidence was found for improved cognitive functions as assessed by the SCAG, but the affective items did demonstrate both active medications to be

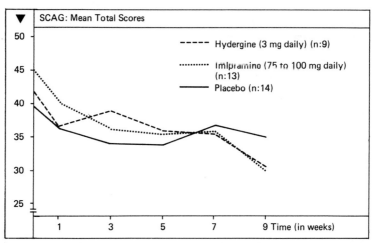

Fig. 9.2. Sandoz Clinical Assessment Geriatric (SCAG) scale total scores: weekly changes in ambulatory older persons with a mild degree of mood and cognitive impairment. (Reproduced with permission from Shader and Goldsmith (1976).)

effective. SCAG cluster scores revealed that only the cluster mood improved significantly when contrasting hydergine and placebo. Statistically significant differences were not observed between the two active treatments.

Gaitz *et al.* (1977) findings demonstrated via the SCAG, the positive effects hydergine has on cognitive dysfunctions. They examined whether hydergine had an independent effect on cognitive dysfunction as opposed to mood depression alone. Multivariate analysis of variance and analysis of covariance showed improvement in both factors, and indicated that changes in cognitive dysfunction cannot be accounted for as a mere reflection associated with improved mood and a general sense of well-being. These findings, however, were not supported by the results obtained on an objective measurement, a mental status checklist. Chudnovsky (1979) also assessed the effects of hydergine in elderly outpatients over a period of six months. Evaluations of study results revealed that only the factors, 'mood depression' and 'interpersonal relationships', significantly improved in contrast to placebo.

Effects on mood and cognitive functions

Thus by organizing the SCAG into different factors one gains a better understanding of treatment efficacy. The above mentioned findings support more the concept the efficacy of hydergine is primarily as a mood elevator but do not substantiate the notion that hydergine consistently improved cognitive functions. Furthermore, it cannot be overlooked that the SCAG is an observer-rating instrument and not an objective measurement of cognitive functions. These points, plus the fact that there is a shortage of objective evidence demonstrating that hydergine improves cognitive functioning in aging and dementia patients, suggest that improvements in these areas are more of a reflection or a result of improved mood and general sense of well-being.

Further support of this notion is provided by Yesavage *et al.* (1981) who reported on the usefulness of hydergine combined with cognitive training (CT) designed to enhance memory and other intellectual functions, by the teaching of organizational schemes and mnemonic devices, in comparison with hydergine plus supportive counselling (SC). They hypothesized that the positive effect of hydergine on affect, would facilitate the learning of psychological methods (CT) to improve memory, and the overall influence of treatment on cognition may be greater than from the drug combined with SC. The results demonstrated a superior effect on memory in the hydergine plus CT group when compared to the hydergine plus SC group. Despite the fact that there was no placebo group, the results provide hope that the combination approach will have more impact than either treatment alone.

Another relevant concern deals with the long-term benefit of hydergine. Eighteen of the studies presented graphs or tables addressing the time-response curves and analyses for key symptoms and/or global ratings, of both treatment groups. Characteristic of the time-response patterns of the hydergine-treated patients was a course of continuing improvement throughout the trial. The curves of the patients in the placebo or papaverine groups, on the other hand, indicated a similar pattern for the first four to six weeks, then they remained unchanged for the duration of the trial or began to regress. These patterns were typical for most of the studies using a 12-week study period, i.e. the placebo effect peaks at around the fifth to sixth week, whereas the hydergine effect continues to reflect improvement.

As mentioned earlier, four studies had longer periods of observation. Gaitz *et al.* (1977) reported on their 24-week study that at the mid-point there was less distinction between the hydergine and placebo group, but after 24 weeks significant differences were noted (Fig. 9.3). The authors suggested that a placebo effect

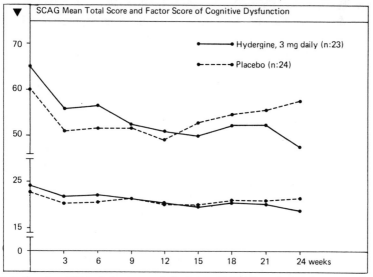

Fig. 9.3. Sandoz Clinical Assessment Geriatric (SCAG) scale total scores: changes over 24 weeks in nursing home residents with evidence of organic brain syndrome. (Data from study of Gaitz *et al.* (1977).)

was quite pronounced until the twelfth week, but that it did not persist over an extended period of time. Soni and Soni (1975), however, communicated in their nine-month study that the most rapid improvement was observed in the first three months, and afterwards the differences were considerably reduced. They indicated that the longer the study is conducted the less significant is the improvement attributable to hydergine. They concluded that hydergine is a valuable drug, but the lack of sustained improvement after three months is disturbing. The longest DB trial covered a span of 15 months (Kugler *et al.* 1978). After six months of treatment differences on the various psychometric performance measures were not significant. After 15 months, however, there was an increase of 5 to 7 per cent in general intelligence (measured by Wechsler Intelligence Test, German version; Dahl 1972) in the hydergine group, whereas in the placebo group there was an 8 per cent decrease in general intelligence. Cerebral circulation time decreased in the hydergine group during the course of the study by 1.3 seconds and in the placebo group increased by 1.5 seconds. EEG changes supported the direction of these time changes.

Another query posed concerns the differential and/or optimal dosage of hydergine. As indicated, the daily dosage in 25 studies was 3 mg and in 13 studies it was 4.5 mg. Yesavage *et al.* (1979) imply, based upon their review of 22 well-controlled studies, that 'trials at the highest dosage (up to 4.5 mg/day) claim the best results, which is consistent with the uncertain absorption of dihydroergotoxin' (Yesavage *et al.* 1979, p. 221). This conclusion, however, was not supported by a DB study involving 14 patients with senile dementia (Yesavage *et al.* 1979). Two dosages, 3 mg and 6 mg daily, were studied in a cross-over method for 24 weeks (12 weeks per treatment) and results revealed little evidence for the superiority of the 6 mg over the 3 mg dosage in the severely impaired sample studied. Based on this review there is no clear-cut evidence favouring the 4.5 mg dosage over the 3 mg. Apparently the higher dosage is more common in Europe.

In summary, there is ample evidence demonstrating the statistical superiority of hydergine over the comparison substance. Areas most responsive to treatment, according to clinicians' ratings, were cognitive dysfunctions and mood-depression. Improvement in cognitive functions, however, was not substantiated by psychometric testing. Such observations, also alluded to by others (Cole 1980; Funkenstein *et al.* 1981; Reisberg *et al.* 1980; Wittenborn 1981), suggest that a positive by-product of improved mood and general sense of well-being might be improvement in cognitive functions. Needed, therefore, are additional clinical trials designed to demonstrate the effects which hydergine has on cognitive functions, as measured by objective psychometric tests; also needed are trials of hydergine in comparison with antidepressants now on the market.

PIRACETAM

Piracetam (2-oxo-1-pyrolidine acetamide) is a cyclic derivative of gamma-aminobutyric acid (GABA). Claims are made that it is possible with piracetam to enhance, directly and preferentially, the efficiency of the telencephalic integrative activities. Telencephalic integrative activity of the brain is defined tentatively as:

'the body of operations through which the brain accomplishes its most specific function, i.e. enables us to acquire new experiences, to retrieve past ones, and by a constant interaction between them to interfere with our own past and future' (Giurgea 1976, pp. 223-4). These claims are based on the following observations of piracetam in several animal species: Piracetam (i) protects against anoxia; (ii) improves learning and memory in normal and deficient animals in a variety of experimental models; (iii) facilitates interhemispheric transfer of information; and (iv) does not have any effect on behavioural arousal or on the autonomic nervous system (Giurgea 1976, p. 265).

Piracetam is considered to be representative of a new class of pharmacological agents known as nootropics (from *noo* = mind, and *tropein* = toward). Such substances act specifically on the associative, integrative mechanisms of the brain, which leads to a direct, positive effect upon mental function (Giurgea 1976). Such reasoning has resulted in a number of double-blind piracetam studies designed to determine its usefulness in improving functioning in patients with varying degrees of senile dementia. Table 9.6 presents an overview of 13 double-blind piracetam studies.

Methodology of studies

Patients in most of the samples were described as displaying symptoms of mild to moderate dementia, and all but three of the samples consisted of inpatients or nursing-home residents. In total, 881 patients were enrolled in these studies and an equal percentage received either active treatment or placebo. The age of the samples ranged from 54 to 85 years, and pooled together the mean age was 70.3, N:736 (based upon data given for 10 studies). Approximately 60 per cent of the patients were females. Five of the studies were conducted with a cross-over design, whereas the other eight had parallel treatment groups. The daily dosage in the various studies was either 2.4 g (N:7), 3.6 g (N:1), 4.8 g (N:4), or 7.2 g (N:1). In each instance the comparison substance was placebo. The length of investigation extended from a minimum of four weeks (N:5) up to a period of 12 weeks (N:1) with the most common being six weeks (N:6). Clinical rating scales were chosen most often (N:11) to determine efficacy, and psychometric tests were performed in seven trials. Physiological measurements, EEG and CBF, were assessed in two studies (Trabant *et al.* 1977; Gustafson *et al.* 1978, respectively).

Results with piracetam

Seven investigators (Abuzzahab *et al.* 1977; Dencker and Lindberg 1977; Ferris *et al.* 1981; Gustafson *et al.* 1978; Kretschmar and Kretschmar 1976 (low dose); Lloyd-Evans *et al.* 1979; Trabant *et al.* 1977) reported no significant changes (except due to possible random variations), in contrast with placebo, on behavioural rating scales, psychometric tests, and physiological parameters. Reasons cited for this lack of differentiation between treatment groups were: (i) patients were too impaired and no longer had the resources for clinical responses; (ii) the period of observation was too short and the dosage too low. The outcome of the one study in which the period of observation was extended to 12 weeks, however,

TABLE 9.6. Summary of the piracetam studies

Author(s)	Year	Setting	N	$\bar{x}$ age	Piracetam daily doses	Comparison substance	Duration (weeks)	†Results			
								Rating scale	Psychometry	Physiology	Global rating
Abuzzahab et al.	1977	Hospital	56	–	2.4 g	Placebo	8	1/18	0/14	–	S
Dencker and Lindberg	1977	Hospital	30	78	2.4 g	Placebo	6	0/12	0/3	–	–
Dorn	1978	–	42	54	4.8 g	Placebo	4/4	8/20	–	–	–
Ferris et al.	1981	Outpatients	40	–	7.2 g	Placebo	4/4	–	0/10	–	–
Gustafson et al.	1978	Hospital	8	62	4.8/9.6 g	Placebo	4/4/4	0/15	0/6	CBF-NS	–
Kartin et al.	1979	Hospital	57	–	3.6 g	Placebo	4	4/15	–	–	–
Kretschmar and Kretschmar*	1976	Hospital	178	71	2.4 g	Placebo	6	0/20	–	–	NS
	1976	Hospital	78	73	4.8 g	Placebo	6	11/20	–	–	S
Lloyd-Evans et al.	1979	Old age home	78	80	2.4 g	Placebo	12/12	NS	1/14	–	NS
Mindus et al.	1976	Volunteers	18	56	4.8 g	Placebo	4/4	–	7/9	–	–
Parrisius	1977	Old age home	60	83	2.4 g	Placebo	6	S	–	–	S
Stegink	1972	Outpatients	196	67	2.4 g	Placebo	8	4/12	–	–	S
Trabant et al.	1977	Hospital	40	58	2.4 g	Placebo	6	1/13	0/4	EEG-NS	–

*Presented findings on two studies.
†Listed are the number of variables which showed a significant improvement, $p \leqslant 0.05$, in the Piracetam group in comparison with the placebo group.

demonstrated that piracetam was no better than placebo in preventing the progression of dementia in old people (Lloyd-Evans *et al.* 1979). Regarding dosage, it is shown in Table 9.6 that in five of the seven studies from which no significant changes were reported, the lowest dosage of 2.4 g per day was indeed used. In contrast, four of the six investigators who obtained significant differences (Dorn 1978; Kartin *et al.* 1979; Kretschmar and Kretschmar, Study II 1976; Mindus *et al.* 1976), utilized a higher dosage regimen. Nevertheless, Ferris *et al.* (1981) and Gustafson *et al.* (1978) failed to observe significant, positive effects with 7.2 g or 9.6 g of piracetam per day, respectively.

Significant positive effects were observed sporadically in the areas of somatic functioning, cognitive dysfunctions, affect, and overall impression. Dorn (1978) noted improvement in a sample of patients with signs of premature biological aging, in somatic, psychic, and performance measures. It is of interest that patients were selected only if they reacted positively on piracetam during a preliminary six weeks open trial. Kartin *et al.* (1979) studied a group of patients suffering from a recent cerebrovascular accident and observed improvement in motor hypoactivity, apathy, spontaneous activity, and general condition. It was concluded that piracetam facilitates rapid rehabilitation among patients with subacute cerebrovascular accidents.

Kretschmar and Kretschmar (1976) considered the dose–effect relationship of piracetam and found marked improvement with 4.8 g per day in the areas of fatigue, affect, concentration, emotional lability, as well as in terms of global impression. Mindus *et al.* (1976) examined the same dosage with a sample of volunteers and reported improvement on a variety of performance, cognitive, and global variables. It was concluded that even though the results indicated a beneficial effect of piracetam on mental performance in aging, non-deteriorated subjects, it needs to be stressed that the size of the effect was moderate.

Similar trends were reported earlier by Steginck (1972) who treated a large sample of outpatients with piracetam. In contrast to placebo-treated patients, those receiving active substance manifested significant improvement in psychomotor agitation, asthenia, alertness, and overall impression. In the oldest sample studied, and inpatients having reduced cerebral functional capacity, there was evidence of benefitting from 2.4 g of piracetam per day. Results showed a significant reduction in the sum of symptoms in the piracetam-treated group, and likewise the distribution of improved cases was more pronounced (Parrisius 1977).

The composite picture of the reviewed literature suggests that the findings in humans are equivocal, a conclusion also reached in other reviews (Ordy *et al.* 1981; Wittenborn 1981). Favourable results have been reported for young volunteers in terms of increases in short-term memory for words and improved interhemispheric transfer of verbal information (Dimond 1976; Dimond and Brouwers 1976), and also for older healthy volunteers on performance measures (Lagergren and Levander 1974; Mindus *et al.* 1976). These findings have not been substantially replicated with patients suffering from various degrees of dementia. It appears that the claims made on the potential of piracetam in alleviating or inhibiting the cognitive and emotional impairments associated with senile dementia, are not supported by the double-blind piracetam trials reviewed here.

CONCLUSIONS

The chapter presents a comprehensive review of two gerontopsychopharmacological compounds, hydergine and piracetam. In total, 38 double-blind hydergine studies and 13 double-blind piracetam studies were critically examined.

Owing to the similarity of assessment procedures used in the hydergine studies it was easier to examine and identify the behavioural factors which were more responsive. In short, symptoms of cognitive dysfunction and mood-depression were reported as significantly improved, following hydergine therapy. There was also evidence to demonstrate that, over time, patients continue to manifest some degree of improvement. It is suggested that the beneficial effects of hydergine are primarily affective. The findings regarding piracetam, on the other hand, did not support the notion that it is beneficial in alleviating or inhibiting cognitive or emotional impairments associated with senile dementia.

Acknowledgements

I thank Eleonore Kaps for her skill and care in editing and typing this manuscript. I also thank Shering AG and Reinhard Horowski for supporting this work.

REFERENCES

Abuzzahab, F. S., Merwin, G. E., Zimmermann, R. L., and Sherman, M. C. (1977). A double blind investigation of piracetam (Nootropil) vs placebo in geriatric memory. *Pharmakopsychiat.* 10, 49–56.
Anastasi, A. (1976). *Psychological testing*, 4th edn. MacMillian, New York.
Arrigo, A., Braun P., Kauchtschischwili, G. M., Moglia, A., and Tartara, A. (1973). Influence of treatment on symptomatology and correlated electroencephalographic (EEG) changes in the aged. *Curr. Ther. Res.* 15, 417–26.
Ban, T. A. (1980). *Psychopharmacology for the aged.* Karger, Basel.
Banen, D. M. (1972). An ergot preparation (Hydergine) for relief of symptoms of cerebrovascular insufficiency. *J. Am. geriat. Soc.* 20, 22–4.
Bargheon, J. (1973). Etitude on double insu de l'hydergine chez le sujet age. *Nouv. Presse Med.* 2, 2053–5.
Bazo, A. J. (1973). An ergot alkaloid preparation (Hydergine) versus Papaverine in treating common complaints of the aged. Double-blind study. *J. Am. geriat. Soc.* 21, 65–71.
Biel, M.-L., Seus, R., and Struppler, A. (1976). Medikamentöse Therapie des hirnorganischen Psychosyndroms im Alter. *Med. Klin.* 71, 2177–84.
Bochner, F., Eadie, M. J., and Tyrer, J. H. (1973). Use of an ergot preparation (Hydergine) in the convalescent phase of stroke. *J. Am. geriat. Soc.* 21, 10–17.
Botwinick, J. (1973). *Aging and behavior.* Springer, New York.
Branconnier, R. J. and Cole, J. O. (1978). The impairment index as a symptom-independent parameter of drug efficacy in geriatric psychopharmacology. *J. Geront.* 33, 217–23.
Butler, R. N. (1975). *Why survive? Being old in America.* Harper and Row, New York.
— and Lewis, M. A. (1977). *Aging and mental health: positive psychosocial approaches*, 2nd edn. Mosby, St. Louis.

Chudnovsky, N. (1979). Community-based management of mild to moderate mental deterioration in older age outpatients. Scientific exhibit, *American Academy of Family Physicians*, 31st Annual Scientific Assembly, Atlanta, Georgia.

Cole, J. O. (1980). Drug therapy of senile organic brain syndromes. *Psychiat. J. Univ. Ottawa* 5, 41–52.

Corso, J. F. (1977). Auditory perception and communication. In *Handbook of the psychology of aging* (ed. J. E. Birren and K. W. Schaie) pp. 535–53. Van Nostrand Reinhold, New York.

Cox, J. R., Pandurangi, V. R., and Wallace, M. G. (1978). Drugs will help if dementing patients are caught early. *Modern Geriat.* 12–15.

Crook, T. H. (1979). Psychometric assessment in the elderly. In *Psychiatric symptoms and cognitive loss in the elderly* (ed. Raskin, A. and L. F. Jarvik). pp. 207–20. Wiley, New York.

— Ferris, S., Sathananthan, G., Raskin, A., and Gershon, S. (1977). The effect of methylphenidate in test performance in the cognitively impaired aged. *Psychopharmacology* 52, 251–5.

Dahl, G. (1972). *WIP – Reduzierter Wechsler Intelligenz Test.* Verlag Anton Hain, Meisenheim am Glan.

Dencker, S. J. and Lindberg, D. (1977). A controlled double-blind study of piracetam in the treatment of senile dementia. *Nord. Psykiatr. Tidskr.* 31, 48–52.

Dennler, H.-J. and Bachmann, H. (1979). Behandlung der zerebrovaskulären Insuffizienz. *Münch. med. Wschr.* 121, 1615–18.

Derogatis, L. R., Klerman, G. L., and Lipman, R. S. (1972). Anxiety states and depressive neuroses: issues in nosological discrimination. *J. nerv. ment. Dis.* 155, 392–403.

Dimond, S. J. (1976). Drugs to improve learning in man: implications and neuropsychological analysis. In *The neuropsychology of learning disorders* (ed. R. M. Knights, and D. J. Baker) pp. 367–79), University Park Press, Baltimore.

— and Brouwers, E. Y. M. (1976). Increase in the power of human memory in normal man through the use of drugs. *Psychopharmacology* 49, 307–9.

Ditch, M., Kelly, F. J., and Resnik, O. (1971). An ergot preparation (Hydergine) in the treatment of cerebrovascular disorders in the geriatric patient: double-blind study. *J. Am. geriat. Soc.* 19, 208–17.

Dorn, M. (1978). Piracetam bei vorzeitiger biologischer Alterung. *Fortschr. Med.* 96, 1525–30.

Einspruch, B. C. (1976). Helping to make the final years meaningful for the elderly residents of nursing homes. *Dis. nerv. Syst.* 37, 439–42.

Eisdorfer, C. (1968). Arousal and performance: experiments in verbal learning and a tentative theory. In *Human aging and behavior* (ed. G. A. Talland) pp. 189–216. Academic Press, New York.

Ferris, S., Reisberg, B., Crook, T., Friedman, E., Schneck, M., Mir, P., Sherman, K., Corwin, J., Gershon, S., and Bartus, R. (1981). Pharmacology treatment of senile dementia: choline, L-Dopa, Piracetam, and choline plus Piracetam. In *Alzheimer's disease: a report of progress in research* (ed. S. Corkin, K. Davis, J. Growdon, E. Usdin, and R. Wurtman) Vol. 19. Raven Press, New York.

— Sathananthan, G., Gershon, S., and Clark, C. (1977). Senile dementia: treatment with deanol. *J. Am. geriat. Soc.* 35, 240–4.

Food and Drug Commision Reports, 22 October 1979.

Fozard, J. L., Wolf, E., Bell, B., McFarland, R. A., and Podolsky, S. (1977). Visual perception and communication. In *Handbook of the psychology of aging.* (ed. J. E. Birren and K. W. Schaie) pp. 497–534. Van Nostrand Reinhold, New York.

Funkenstein, H. H., Hicks, R., Dysken, M. W., and Davis, J. M. (1981). Drug treatment of cognitive impairment in Alzheimer's disease and the late life dementias. In *Drug treatment of cognitive impairment in Alzheimer's disease and the late life dementias* (ed. N. E. Miller and G. D. Cohen) Vol. 15, pp. 139–60. Raven Press, New York.

Furry, C. A. and Baltes, P. B. (1973). The effect of age differences in ability – extraneous performance variables on the assessment of intelligence in children, adults, and the elderly. *J. Geront.* **28**, 73–80.

Gaitz, Ch. M., Varner, R. V., and Overall, J. E. (1977). Organic brain syndrome in late life. *Archs gen. Psychiat.* **34**, 839–47.

Gauron, E. F. and Dickinson, J. K. (1969). The influence of seeing the patient first on diagnostic decision making in psychiatry. *Am. J. Psychiat.* **126**, 199–205.

Gerin, J. (1969). Treatment of cerebrovascular insufficiency with Hydergine. *Curr. ther. Res.* **11**, 539–46.

Giurgea, C. (1976). Piracetam: nootropic pharmacology of neurointegrative activity. In *Current developments in psychopharmacology* (ed. W. B. Essman and L. Valzelli) Vol. 3, pp. 221–74. Spectrum, New York.

Gottschalk, L. A. (1975). Drug effects in the assessment of affective states in man. In *Current developments in psychopharmacology* (ed. W. B. Essman and L. Valzelli) Vol. 1, pp. 261–99. Spectrum, New York.

Grill, P. and Broicher, H. (1969). Zur Therapie der zerebralen Insuffizienz. *Dt. med. Wschr.* **94**, 2429–35.

Gurland, B. I. (1980). The assessment of the mental health status of older adults. In *Handbook of mental health and aging* (ed. J. E. Birren and R. B. Sloan) pp. 671–700. Prentice-Hall, New York.

Gustafson, L., Risberg, J., Johanson, M., Fransson, M., and Maximilian, V. A. (1978). Effects of Piracetam on regional cerebral blood flow and mental functions in patients with organic dementia. *Psychopharmacology* **56**, 115–17.

Heiss, R., Seus, R., and Fahrenberg, J. (1969). Eine Studie zur Prüfung der psychodynamischen Wirkung von Dihydroergotoxin. *Arzneim.-Forsch.* **21**, 797–800.

Herzfeld, U., Christian, W., Oswald, W. D., Ronge, J., and Wittgen, M. (1972). Zur Wirkungsanalyse von Hydergin im Langzeitversuch. *Med. Klin.* **67**, 1118–25.

Hicks, R., Funkenstein, H., Davis, J., and Dysken, M. (1980). Geriatric psychopharmacology. In *Handbook of mental health and aging* (ed. J. E. Birren and R. B. Sloane) pp. 745–74. Prentice-Hall, New York.

Hollingsworth, S. W. (1980). Response of geriatric patients from the satellite nursing homes of Maricopa Country to hydergine therapy: a double-blind study. *Curr. Ther. Res.* **27**, 401–10.

Honigfeld, G. (1982). The evaluation of ward behavior rating scales for psychogeriatric use. *Psycholpharm. Bull.* **17**, 81–95.

Hughes, J. R., Williams, J. G., and Currier, R. D. (1976). An ergot alkaloid preparation (Hydergine) in the treatment of dementia: critical review of the clinical literature. *J. Am. geriat. Soc.* **24**, 490–7.

Jennings, W. G. (1972). An ergot alkaloid preparation (Hydergine) versus placebo for treatment of symptoms of cerebrovascular insufficiency: double-blind study. *J. Am. geriat. Soc.* **20**, 407–12.

Kahn, R. L., Zarit, S. H., Hilbert, N. M., and Niederehe, G. (1975). Memory complaints and impairment in the aged. *Archs gen. Psychiat.* **32**, 1569–73.

Karasu, T. B., Stein, S. P., and Charles, E. S. (1979). Age factors in patient-therapist relationship. *J. nerv. ment. Dis.* **167**, 100–4.

Kartin, P., Povse, M., and Skondia, V. (1979). Clinical study of Piracetam in patients with subacute cerebrovascular accidents. *Acta ther.* **5**, 235–43.

Katz, M. M., Cole, J. O., and Lowery, H. A. (1969). Studies of the diagnostic process: the influence of symptom perception, past experience, and ethnic background on diagnostic decisions. *Am. J. Psychiat.* **125**, 937–47.

Kochansky, G. F. (1979). Psychiatric rating scales for assessing psychopathology in the elderly. In *Psychiatric symptoms and cognitive loss in the elderly* (ed. A. Raskin and L. F. Jarvik) pp. 125–56. Wiley, New York.

Kramer, N. A. and Jarvik, L. F. (1979). Assessment of intellectual changes in the elderly. In *Psychiatric symptoms and cognitive loss in the elderly. Evaluation and assessment techniques* (ed. A. Raskin and L. F. Jarvik) pp. 221–72. Wiley, New York.

Kretschmar, J. H. and Kretschmar, C. (1976) Zur Dosis-Wirkungs-Relation bei der Behandlung mit Piracetam. *Arzneim.-Forsch.* **26**, 1153–7.

Kugler, J., Oswald, W. D., Herzfeld, U., Seus, R., Pingel, J., and Welzel, D. (1978). Langzeittherapie altersbedingter Insuffizienzerscheinungen des Gehirns. *Dt. med. Wschr.* **103**, 456–62.

Lagergren, K. and Levander, S. A. (1974). A double-blind study on the effects of piracetam upon perceptual and psychomotor performance at varied heart rates in patients treated with artificial pacemakers. *Psychopharmacologia* **39**, 97–104.

Lezak, M. D. (1976). *Neuropsychological assessment.* Oxford University Press, New York.

Lifschitz, K. (1960). Problems in the quantitative evaluation of patients with psychoses of the senium. *J. Psychol.* **49**, 295.

Linden, M. E. (1975). Retirement and the elderly patient – problems and practical therapy. Scientific exhibit, *32nd Annual Meeting of the American Geriatrics Society*, Miami Beach, Florida.

Lloyd-Evans, S., Brocklehurst, J. C., and Palmer, M. K. (1978). Assessment of drug therapy in chronic brain failure. *Gerontology* **24**, 304–11.

— — — (1979). Piracetam in chronic brain failure. *Curr. med. Res. Opin.* **6**, 351–7.

Loew, D. M. (1980). Pharmacologic approaches to the treatment of senile dementia. In *Aging of the brain and dementia* (ed. L. Amaducci, A. N. Davison, and P. Antuono) *Aging* Vol. 13, pp. 287–94. Raven Press, New York.

— and Vigouret, J. M. (1981). Pharmacologic approaches to gerontopsychiatry. In *Handbook of experimental pharmacology* (ed. F. Hoffmeister and G. Stille) No. 55, Vol. 2, pp. 435–60. Springer, Berlin.

— —and Jaton, A. L. (1979). Effects of dihydroergotoxine mesylate (Hydergine[R]) on cerebral synaptic transmission. *Interdisc. top. Geront.* **15**, 85–103.

McConnachie, R. W. (1973). A clinical trial comparing 'Hydergine' with placebo in the treatment of cerebrovascular insufficiency in elder patients. *Curr. med. Res. Opin.* **1**, 463–8;

— (1978). The clinical assessment of brain failure in the elderly. *Pharmacology* **16** Suppl. 1, 27–35.

McDonald, R. J. (1979). Hydergine: a review of 26 clinical studies. *Pharmakopsychiat* **12**, 407–22.

— and Suchy, I. (1980). Der Einfluss subjectiver Beschwerden auf Leistung und Befindlichkeit im Alter. *Z. Geront.* **13**, 346–58.

Markstein, R. and Wagner, H. (1978). Effect of dihydroergotoxine on cyclic AMP-generating systems in rat cerebral cortex slices. *Gerontology* Suppl. 1, **24**, 94–105.

Matejcek, M. (1980). Cortical correlates of vigilance regulation and their use in evaluating the effects of treatment. In *Ergot compounds and brain function: neuroendocrine and neuropsychiatric aspects* (ed. M. Goldstein, A. Lieberman, D. B. Calne, and M. O. Thorner) pp. 339–48. Raven Press, New York.

— Knor, K., Piguet, P., and Weil, C. (1979). Electroencephalographic and clinical changes as correlated in geriatric patients treated three months with an ergot alkaloid preparation. *J. Am. geriat. Soc.* **27**, 198–202.

Meier-Ruge, W., Emmenegger, H., Enz, A., Gygax, P., Iwangoff, P., and Wiernsperger, N. (1978). Pharmacological aspects of dihydrogenated ergot alkaloids in experimental brain research. *Pharmacology* Suppl. 1, **16**, 45–62.

— Enz, A., Gygax, P., Hunziker, O., Iwangoff, P., and Reichlmeier, K. (1975). Experimental pathology in basic research of the aging brain. In *Genesis and treatment of psychologic disorders in the elderly* (ed. S. Gershon and A. Raskin) Vol. 2, pp. 55–126. Raven Press, New York.

Miller, E. (1980). Cognitive assessment of the older adult. In *Handbook of mental health* (ed. I. E. Birren and R. B. Sloane) pp. 520–36. Prentice-Hall, New York.

— (1981). The differential psychological evaluation. In *Clinical aspects of Alzheimer's disease and senile dementia* (ed. E. Miller and G. Cohen) Vol. 15, pp. 121–36. Raven Press, New York.

Mindus, P., Cornholm, B., Levander, S. E., and Schalling, D. (1976). Piracetam-induced improvement of mental performance. *Acta psychiat. scand.* **54**, 150–60.

Mongeau, B. (1974). The effect of Hydergine on the transit time of cerebral circulation in diffuse cerebral insufficiency. *Eur. J. clin. Pharmac.* **7**, 169–75.

Nelson, J. J. (1975). Relieving select symptoms of the elderly. *Geriatrics* **30**, 133–42.

Nicrosini, F. and Pasotti, C. (1976). Studio clinico controllato sull' attivita e sulla tollerabilita del Trivastan. *Min. Med.* **67**, 1745–50.

Ordy, J. M., Brizzee, K. R., and Bartus, R. T. (1981). Neuropsychopharmacology: drug modification of memory in relation to aging in human and nonhuman primate brain. In *Clinical Pharmacology and the aged patient* (ed. L. F. Jarvik, D. J. Greenblatt, and D. Harman) *Aging* Vol. 16, pp. 79–102, Raven Press, New York.

Oswald, W. D. (1979). Psychometrische Verfahren und Fragebogen für gerontopsychologische Untersuchungen. *Z. Geront.* **12**, 341–50.

— and Lang, E. (1980). Therapeutische Beeinflussung von Leistung und Selbstbild bei geriatrischen Patienten. *Münch. med. Wschr.* **122**, 59–62.

Parrisius, H. W. (1977). Doppelblindstudie mit Piracetam in der Geriatrie. *Geriatrie* **7**, 32–7.

Pfeiff, E., Schlegel, H.-E., Seus, R., Dennler, H. J., and Kugler, J. (1980). Therapie des hirnorganischen Psychosyndroms mit Hydergin und Digitalis. *Med. Welt* **31**, 1403–7.

Rabbit, P. M. A. (1965). An age-decrement in the ability to ignore irrelevant information. *J. Geront.* **20**, 233–8.

Rao, D. B. and Norris, J. R. (1972). A double-blind investigation of Hydergine in the treatment of cerebrovascular insufficiency in the elderly. *Johns Hopkins med. J.* **130**, 317–24.

Rehmann, S. A. (1973). Two trials comparing 'Hydergine' with placebo in the treatment of patients suffering from cerebrovascular insufficiency. *Curr. med. Res. Opin.* **1**, 456–61.

Reisberg, B. (1981). Metabolic enhancers and agents effecting blood flow and oxygen utilization. In *Strategies for the development of an effective treatment for senile dementia* (ed. T. Crook and S. Gershon). Mark Prowley Associates.

— Ferris, S. H., and Gershon, S. (1980). Pharmacotherapy of senile dementia. In *Psychopathology in the aged* (ed. J. O. Cole and J. E. Barret) pp. 233–64. Raven Press, New York.

Rosen, H. J. (1975). Mental decline in the elderly: pharmacotherapy (ergot alkaloids versus papaverine). *J. Am. geriat. Soc.* **23**, 169–74.

Roubicek, J., Geiger, C., and Abt, K. (1972). An ergot alkaloid preparation (Hydergine) in geriatric therapy. *J. Am. geriat. Soc.* **20**, 222–9.
Salzman, C., Kochansky, G. E., and Shader, R. I. (1972). Rating scales for geriatric psychopharmacology. *Psychopharmac. Bull.* **8**, 3–50.
Savage, R. D., Britton, P. G., Bolton, N., and Hall, E. H. (1973). *Intellectual functioning in the aged.* Harper and Row, New York.
Schaie, K. W. (ed.) (1968). *Theory and methods of research on aging.* West Virginia University, Morgantown.
Shader, R. I. and Goldsmith, G. N. (1976). Dihydrogenated ergot alkaloids and papaverine: a status report of their effects in senile mental deterioration. In *Progress in psychiatric treatment* (ed. D. F. Klein and R. Gittelman-Klein) Vol. 2, pp. 540–55. Brunner/Mazel, New York.
— Harmatz, J. S., and Salzman, C. (1974). A new scale for clinical assessment in geriatric populations: Sandoz Clinical Assessment-Geriatric (SCAG). *J. Am. geriat. Soc.* **22**, 107–13.
— — and Tammerk, H.-A. (1979). Towards an observation structure for rating dysfunction and pathology in ambulatory geriatrics. In *CNS aging and its neuropharmacology* (ed. W. Meier-Ruge) Vol. 15, pp. 153–68. Karger, Basel.
Short, M. J. and Benway, M. (1972). *Delivery of mental health services to the elderly . . . the State Hospital and the community.* American Psychiatric Association, Texas.
Singer, J. and Hamot, H. (1980). Problems and opportunities in geriatric clinical trial methodology after a decade of research. *Proc. Int. Cerebrovasc. Dis.* pp. 337–43.
Soni, S. D. and Soni, S. S. (1975). Dihydrogenated alkaloids of ergotoxine in non-hospitalised elderly patients. *Curr. med. Res. Opin.* **3**, 464–8.
SteginK, A. J. (1972). The clinical use of Piracetam, a new nootropic drug. *Arzneim.-Forsch.* **22**, 975–7.
Thibault, A. (1974). A double-blind evaluation of 'Hydergine' and placebo in the treatment of patients with organic brain syndrome and cerebral arteriosclerosis in a nursing home. *Curr. med. Res. Opin.* **2**, 482–7.
Trabant, R., Poljakovic, Z., and Trabant, D. (1977). Zur Wirkung von Piracetam auf das hirnorganische Psychosyndrom bei zerebrovaskulärer Insuffizienz. *Ther. Gegenwart* **116**, 1504–21.
Triboletti, F. and Ferri, H. (1969). Hydergine for treatment of symptoms of cerebrovascular insufficiency. *Curr. ther. Res.* **11**, 609–20.
Venn, R. D. (1978). Clinical pharmacology of ergot alkaloids in senile cerebral insufficiency. In *Ergot alkaloids and related compounds* (ed. B. Berde and H. O. Schild) pp. 533–66. Springer, Berlin.
Wechsler, D. (1945). A standardized memory scale for clinical use. *J. Psychol.* **19**, 87–95.
— (1955). *Manual for the Wechsler Adult Intelligence Scale.* The Psychology Corporation.
Welford, A. (1976). Motivation, capacity, learning and age. *Int. Aging hum. Devl.* **7**, 189–99.
— (1977). Motor performance. In *Handbook of the psychology of aging* (ed. J.E. Birren and K.W. Schaie) pp. 450–97. Van Nostrand Reinhold, New York.
— (1980). Sensory, perceptual and motor process in older adults. In *Handbook of mental health and aging* (ed. J. E. Birren and R. B. Sloane) pp. 192–213. Prentice-Hall, Englewood Cliffs.
Wells, C. E. and Buchanan, D. C. (1979). The clinical use of psychological testing in evaluation for dementia. In *Dementia* (ed. C. E. Wells) 2nd edn, pp. 189–204. Davis, Philadelphia.
Westreich, G., Alter, M. and Lundgren, S. (1975). The effect of cyclandelate on dementia. *Stroke* **6**, 535–8.

Wilder, B. J. and Gonyea, E. F. (1973). The effects of the dihydrogenated ergot alkaloids on symptoms of aging. Scientific Exhibit of *American Medical Association Annual Convention*, New York.

Wilson, W. P., Musella, L., and Short, M. J. (19??). The electroencephalogram in dementia. In *Dementia* (ed. C. E. Wells) 2nd edn, pp. 205-22. Davis, Philadelphia.

Winslow, I. (1974). The hospitalized geriatric patient. Scientific Exhibit *American Medical Association 28th Clinical Convention*, Oregon.

Wittenborn, J. R. (1967). Do rating scales objectify clinical impression? *Comp. Psychiat.* **8**, 386-92.

—— (1972). Reliability, validity and objectivity of symptom-rating scales. *J. nerv. ment. Dis.* **154**, 79-87.

—— (1981). Pharmacotherapy for age-related behavioral deficiencies. *J. nerv. ment. Dis.* **169**, 139-56.

Yager, J. (1977). Psychiatric eclecticism: a cognitive view. *Am. J. Psychiat.* **134**, 736-41.

Yesavage, J. A., Hollister, L. E., and Burian, E. (1979a). Dihydroergotoxine: 6-mg versus 3-mg dosage in the treatment of senile dementia. Preliminary report. *J. Am. geriat. Soc.* **27**, 80-2.

—— Tinklenberg, J. R., Hollister, L. E., and Berger, P. A. (1979b) Vasodilators in senile dementias. A review of the literature. *Archs gen. Psychat.* **36**, 220-3.

—— Westphal, J., and Rush, L. (1981). Senile dementia: combined pharmacologic and psychologic treatment. *J. Am. geriat. Soc.* **29**, 164-71.

Zawadski, R. T., Glazer, G. B., and Lurie, E. (1978). Psychotropic drug use among institutionalized and noninstutitionalized medicaid aged in California. *J. Geront.* **33**, 824-34.

10

Measurement of change in the elderly

ANTONIA WHITEHEAD

In this Chapter, the main focus will be upon the measurement of change in the confused elderly and/or those with dementia. Three main issues are considered — the choice of what to measure; the psychometric problems inherent in the measurement; and then some possible solutions.

FUNCTIONS TO BE MEASURED

The first question that has to be asked is what would be appropriate to measure. The answer to this might seem obvious but in this choice it is necessary to bear in mind some questions. Supposing a treatment is being applied that it is hoped will be of benefit to dementing people. The first question is whether the processes to be measured are of practical or theoretical relevance. For the dementing individual and his family, improvements in memory function or self-care ability will be of prime importance. Increased sedation thresholds would not be of themselves of any value; but might be of critical importance in attempting to understand the action of the treatment given. The second question to ask is how direct a measurement can be made of the relevant function or ability. It is too easy to fall into the trap of using an indirect measure, which does correlate with level on the function of interest, but unless this correlation is very high indeed, it is unlikely that useful results will be gained in this way, since too many other factors could also influence the level of performance. A third question is whether the function is known to be impaired at this level of dementia. In advanced dementia, it is only too possible to demonstrate impairments on almost all types of ability and capability. However, early on, no impairments would be demonstrable on some commonly used tasks, such as vocabulary knowledge and span of immediate recall (e.g. Whitehead 1973). If an ability is not notably impaired, it is of little value to measure it since improvement with treatment is unlikely.

PSYCHOMETRIC CONSIDERATIONS

The first problem in measuring level of functioning in dementia is to set the difficulty level of the task about right. All too often, material is used that is too difficult for a large proportion of the subjects being tested. This can have a number of unfortunate consequences. When applying a treatment for dementia, there are really four possible outcomes: the patients stay about the same, tend to get better, tend to get worse, or some get better and some get worse. With a proper measurement tool, all these four possibilities can be distinguished from

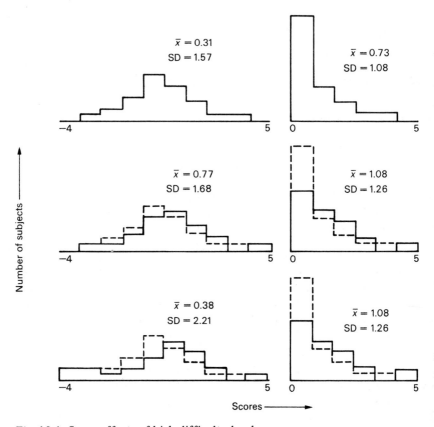

Fig. 10.1 Some effects of high difficulty level

each other. If the range is artificially truncated by using too difficult a task, it is less clear that the consequences can be reliably distinguished. In Fig. 10.1, an attempt has been made to illustrate problems that may arise (the outcome of patients getting worse has been left out for the sake of simplicity).

In Fig. 10.1, the first thing that will be noticed is that the truncation of the range leads to the unfortunate consequence of creating a distribution that is strictly not appropriate for the application of parametric statistics. There are also more subtle problems. In each example, the dotted line illustrates the distribution of scores pretreatment and the solid line that following treatment. In the first example, these coincide; there has been no alteration of scores. In the second case, there is actually a slight improvement; here the truncation conceals this in part and there is a risk that a significant trend towards improvement may fail to be demonstrable on the data remaining. The third case illustrates the outcome where some patients improve while others get worse (a not altogether uncommon finding with what may be termed 'active treatments'). This should lead to the mean level remaining constant while the variance increases. It will be noted that, given the full range of scores, this can be readily seen as different from the case above when there was overall improvement, but where the scores have been truncated the two are indistinguishable. Thus there is a risk that the apparent increase in mean score is taken as showing the treatment as beneficial, since the worsening by some is concealed.

A second major consideration is of the reliability of the measure being used. It has to be noted that scales do not have some absolute reliability level, since this is highly dependent on the type of population being measured; but it is as well to try to choose scales or tests that have previously been shown to have satisfactory levels of reliability on subjects similar to those under consideration.

ASSESSMENT SCALES

I should like to consider a few of the readily available scales that are of about the right difficulty level for dementing subjects. These are by no means all the possible measurement techniques available, nor would they be suitable for all kinds of study. In my choice, I have been guided by an attempt to cover a wide range of different abilities, all of which become impaired at some stage in the dementing process. It must be said that in few of these tasks would it even be pretended to measure 'pure' functions; this would perhaps be an impossible goal in dementia.

The CAPE scale

The first scale I want to consider is the Clifton Assessment Procedure for the Elderly, normally known as the CAPE (Pattie and Gilleard 1979). This has two scales, the Behaviour Rating Scale and the Cognitive Assessment Scale. In Table 10.1 are shown the four subscales of the Behaviour Rating Scale. In all, there are

TABLE 10.1. *Clifton Assessment Procedure for the Elderly (CAPE) behaviour rating scale (psychometric characteristics)*

	Floor (SD)	r^*
Physical disability	1.8	0.85
Apathy	>2	0.87
Communication difficulties	0.8	0.72
Social disturbance	1.1	0.72
Total	>2	–

*Inter-rater reliability.

18 items each rated on a 0-2 scale by someone giving care to the individual. It will be seen that the inter-rater reliability is adequate. The 'floor' of the scale has been estimated by the distance (in standard deviations) between the sample mean and the worst possible score. Ideally, this should be at least 2, since this would allow almost all the sample to gain scores. Again it has to be stressed that such an estimate is entirely dependent on the sample used, and this differs among the various studies that I am illustrating here and in the following paragraphs. The data here are from Pattie and Gilleard (1979) for subjects diagnosed as suffering from dementia. For these, the floor is satisfactorily low.

The other part of the CAPE is the Cognitive Assessment Scale and, as can be

TABLE 10.2. *Clifton Assessment Procedure for the Elderly (CAPE) cognitive assessment scale (psychometric characteristics)*

	Floor (SD)	r*
Information/orientation	1.1	0.87
Mental ability	1.5	0.89
Psychomotor	0.8	0.79
Total	1.4	–

*Over 3–4 days test–retest.

seen in Table 10.2; this consists of three subscales measuring information and orientation, mental ability (which has material such as counting and reading) and psychomotor ability, which requires the subject to draw his way out of a maze as quickly as possible without touching walls or obstructions. Again the reliability (in this case on test-retest) and the floor are adequate for dementing subjects.

Other tasks

Table 10.3 shows a variety of other tasks measuring different abilities. Vocabulary knowledge can be measured using the WAIS Vocabulary. This appears to be less confusing for dementing people than the alternatives, such as the Mill Hill Vocabulary Scale. I do not have test-retest reliability data on this for dementing subjects, but even over one year, for a mixed sample, the correlation between the scores on the two occasions was quite high (Whitehead 1977). The 'floor' was estimated for dementing subjects.

TABLE 10.3. *Other tasks (psychometric characteristics)*

	Floor (SD)	r
WAIS Vocabulary	1.5	0.72*
Inglis Tasks	1.1	0.69*
Object Learning Test	1.2	0.85†
Digit Copying Test	1.9	0.85†
Parietal Scale	1.7	0.70*

*Retest one year later (mixed group).
†Test-retest (six weeks).

PROBLEMS AND SOLUTIONS

The problem with some learning and memory tests is that they are very difficult for dementing subjects and therefore stressful for them, and for that matter for the tester, to complete. My own solution (Whitehead 1976) to this has been to use a task derived from the Inglis Paired Associate Learning Test, which allows each subject to start with material of intermediate difficulty and then progress to more difficult or less difficult material, as is appropriate. This is shown in Table 10.4; the difficulty level is determined by the degree of association between the stimulus and response words.

TABLE 10.4. *Inglis Tasks for paired associates learning*

Hard		Mediate		Easy	
Flower	– Spark	Cup	– Plate	Knife	– Fork
Table	– River	Cat	– Milk	East	– West
Bottle	– Comb	Gold	– Lead	Hand	– Foot

An alternative solution has been put foward by Gibson and Kendrick (1979) in the revised Kendrick Battery. They use an Object Learning Test, which really consists of a variety of Kim's Game with pictures of common objects being shown on a card, and the subject being required to recall as many as he can. An advantage of this test is a parallel form for re-testing. The test–retest correlation using the alternate form is quite high. It will be seen, however, that the 'floor' of both these tests is somewhat high for dementing subjects, despite the attempts to render the material simple.

Speed can be assessed using the Digit Copying Test also from the revised Kendrick Battery. Both test–retest reliability and the 'floor' for this are satisfactory. Parietal lobe function (presumably apraxia and agnosia) can be assessed using the Parietal Scale (McDonald 1969). Reliability data is not available, but over one year the correlation between the two occasions of testing with a mixed group was quite high and the 'floor' for dementing subjects is satisfactory.

A question that has not been touched upon is that of the validity of these estimates of change. Direct evidence is lacking. The two subtests of the Kendrick Battery have been primarily developed for the detection of dementia, rather than as measures of its extent. The CAPE has *inter alia* useful information about suitable residential placement according to level of scores; it may be supposed that changed level might indicate a capacity to cope in a different setting. Changes in the WAIS Vocabulary, Inglis tasks, and the Parietal Scale, over one year, have been studied in a mixed group of elderly patients.

In general, performance tends to improve but it has been demonstrated that a tendency towards decreased scores was associated with an admission diagnosis of chronic brain syndrome (Whitehead 1977). These patients have now been followed for a further four years and it has been found that those who failed to survive for this time, had shown a differential tendency to gain lower scores on the second occasion of testing. These were naturally-occurring changes. The implications of induced changes, which is the question under present consideration, is a matter that can only be answered in the future. Let us hope that this future is not too distant.

REFERENCES

Gibson, A.J. and Kendrick, D.C. (1979). *The Kendrick Battery for the detection of dementia in the elderly*. NFER, Windsor.

McDonald, C. (1969). Clinical heterogeneity in senile dementia. *Br. J. Psychiat.* **115**, 267–71.

Pattie, A.H. and Gilleard, C.J. (1979). *Manual of the Clifton Assessment Procedure for the elderly*. Hodder and Stoughton, Sevenoaks, Kent.

Whitehead, A. (1973). Verbal learning and memory in elderly depressives. *Br. J. Psychiat.* **123**, 203–8.
— (1976). The prediction of outcome in elderly psychiatric patients. *Psychol. Med.* **6**, 469–79.
— (1977). Changes in cognitive functioning in elderly psychiatric patients. *Br. J. Psychiat.* **130**, 605–8.

11

Deafness, dementia, and depression

KATIA R. GILHOME HERBST

This paper reports on the relationship between acquired deafness and organic brain syndrome (dementia) and acquired deafness and depression in the elderly living at home. These findings constitute just some of the results (which are already reported elsewhere) of a recently completed study, whose major objective was to investigate whether the high prevalence of deafness amongst the elderly living at home which was thought to exist, is related to the high prevalence of mental disorders known to exist (Gilhome Herbst and Humphrey 1980, 1981; Gilhome Herbst 1981; Humphrey *et al.* 1981). The study was carried out from the department of applied social studies at the Polytechnic of North London and represents part of the second phase of a six-year programme of research into the social and psychological implications of acquired deafness (Thomas and Gilhome Herbst 1980*a,b*; Harris *et al.* 1981; Thomas and Ring 1981). This particular part of the programme was funded by the Nuffield Foundation.

BACKGROUND TO THE STUDY

The impetus to undertake this investigation arose from two main sources. The first was the finding, in the previous work of myself and my colleagues, that the overriding effect of acquired deafness in adults of employment age was significant unhappiness, loneliness, withdrawal, and depression. Indeed, we estimated that the adventitiously deaf of employment age were four to five times as likely as the normally hearing, to suffer from anxiety and depression (Thomas and Gilhome Herbst 1980). It therefore seemed reasonable to put forward the hypothesis that acquired deafness, insofar as it constitutes one of the many losses associated with the aging process, may contribute to the precipitation of depression in old age as well. No such an association had yet been established on the basis of systematic enquiry.

The second source was the work of two teams of geriatricians investigating the possible social and medical causes of mental disorders in the elderly. Of the many such studies (Cosin *et al.* 1957; Post 1958; Bergmann 1977), only two suggest that deafness may play some part in the development of organic mental disorders.

One team was originally based at the medical school of the university of Newcastle upon Tyne and their original results have been reported (Kay *et al.* 1964*a,b*). The other team conducted their enquiries as part of the anniversary activities of the Royal College of Physicians and have been reported by Hodkinson (1973).

Kay *et al.* estimated that 62 per cent of the elderly in their sample, with organic brain syndrome, were deaf, while only 31 per cent of the mentally normal were deaf, and they therefore concluded that 'It is possible that those defects of sight and hearing may have sometimes played a part in the production of the mental symptoms by reducing the subjects' contact with the outside world; for the association of sensory defects with mental states seemed to be too strong to be wholly explicable by advanced age of the subjects'. This opinion was tentatively supported by Hodkinson, who estimated that in a sample of 588 geriatric inpatients, 52 per cent of the confused, 47.5 per cent of the demented, and 29 per cent of the mentally normal, were hearing impaired.

Audiometry was not used in the assessment of deafness of either team of geriatricians. Nor, evidently, has it been used in the few community studies that have observed a relationship between deafness and depression in the elderly living at home (Goldberg 1970; Charatan 1975; Garland 1978). Indeed, an extensive review of the literature for this present investigation disclosed no previous community-based study which had used audiometric techniques to estimate the prevalence of acquired hearing loss amongst the elderly. Present estimates (employed by the Department of Health and Social Security) are based on the findings of a variety of studies which have either simply asked the elderly respondent whether they had any difficulty with their hearing (Sheldon 1948; Wilkins 1948; Milne 1976; Abrams 1978), or which have relied upon the observations of the clinician or interviewer in charge (Williamson *et al.* 1964; Sheard 1971; Cumbria County Council 1973). These studies consistently suggest that between 30 to 40 per cent of all elderly people living at home are hearing impaired.

We were therefore faced with two major tasks. The first was to systematically assess the presence of acquired deafness in our target population and the second was to assess mental state.

INDIVIDUALS AND METHODS

The sample consisted of all persons aged 70 years or over registered at the central surgery of a group general practice in an Inner London Borough. Sixty-nine per cent of the target population participated – a response rate comparable with other medicosocial studies on elderly persons living in the community (Milne *et al.* 1971). The age and sex profile of those not included in the analysis showed no significant difference between respondents and non-respondents on these measures. The final sample for analysis was 253.

TABLE 11.1. *Age and sex distribution of the sample*

Sex	Age (years) 70–74		75–79		80–84		85+		Total	
	No.	(%)	No.	(%)	No.	(%)	No.	(%)	No.	(%)
Male	46	(41)	34	(46)	7	(20)	5	(16)	92	(36)
Female	66	(59)	40	(54)	28	(80)	27	(84)	161	(64)
Total	112	(100)	74	(100)	35	(100)	32	(100)	253	(100)

From Gilhome Herbst and Humphrey (1981), with permission.

The interview schedule took on average 1½ hours to complete. It was carried out during one home visit to each respondent and comprised five main areas of interest: the assessment of deafness, mental state, loneliness and isolation, general health and physical mobility and general demographic details.

Measuring deafness

Hearing loss was measured using pure-tone audiometry (air conduction) over the speech frequencies at 250 Hz, 500 Hz, 1 kHz, 2 kHz, and 4 kHz for both ears. Masking was considered unnecessary. Audiocups were fitted to the Amplivox 2150 portable diagnostic audiometer used. A history of any hearing impairment, the experience of deafness and use of aids (where applicable) was taken. As a side-effect of this study a total of 44 referrals for hearing aids (19 requiring domiciliary visits) were made direct to the Hearing Aid Centre at the Royal National Throat, Nose and Ear Hospital, London, by prior arrangement.

We were able to analyse the audiogrammes of these persons re-tested under clinical conditions, and so validate our own audiometry performed in the homes of the elderly people. A very high level of agreement (an overall mean difference of 0.3 dB) was found between the average decibel levels of respondents tested at The Royal National Hospital and tested by ourselves in the field.

Mental state

Scales to screen for organic brain syndrome and depression were extracted from the Comprehensive Assessment and Referral Evaluation (CARE) Schedule (Gurland *et al*. 1977). The CARE Schedule is, briefly, an updated version of the Geriatric Mental State Schedule (GMS) (Copeland *et al*. 1976) now deemed suitable for use by non-medical personnel. My colleagues and I were trained to use it at the Institute of Psychiatry, London. During fieldwork, an independent clinical psychiatrist, with experience in research and psychiatry in old age, was appointed to carry out 10 clinical interviews to validate the administration of the measuring device by the research team and a very high level of agreement was found.

RESULTS

Incidence of deafness

As a measure of deafness, the level of impairment where it is normally considered necessary for patients to need a hearing aid (an average loss of 35 dB or more over the speech frequencies at 1 kHz, 2 kHz, and 4 kHz in the better ear) was used. It was established that deafness was present in 60 per cent of those aged 70 years and over, 69 per cent of those aged 75 years and over, 82 per cent of those aged 80 years and over, and 84 per cent of those aged 85 years and over.

There were two other major findings:

1. Deafness increased significantly with age (at the 0.1 per cent level), such that for the older age groups deafness is the *norm* and not the exception.

2. Increased age is significantly related to *severity* of deafness (at the 0.1 per cent level), such that the older you are the more likely you are to be very deaf indeed.

TABLE 11.2. *The relationship between advanced age and degree of deafness*

Degree of deafness	Age (years) 70–79 No. (%)	80+ No. (%)	Total No. (%)
0–34 dB not deaf	88 (47)	12 (18)	100 (40)
35–44 dB 'moderately' deaf	38 (20)	8 (12)	46 (18)
45–69 dB 'substantially' deaf	47 (25)	34 (51)	81 (32)
70 dB+ 'severely' deaf	13 (7)	13 (19)	26 (10)
Total	186 (100)	67 (100)	253 (100)

From Gilhome Herbst and Humphrey (1980), with permission.
χ^2 = 30.09 with 3 d.f. p < 0.001.

TABLE 11.3. *Estimates of prevalence of deafness in the elderly population based on self-assessment by respondents*

Author	Age (years) 60+	65+	70+	75+	80+	85+
Sheldon (1948)	29%F	38%M	–	–	–	60%M 68%F
Wilkins (1948)	–	–	–	28%M 25%F	–	–
Harris (1962)	–	35%M 30%F	–	–	–	–
Kay *et al.* (1964*a*,*b*)	–	37%	–	–	–	–
Richardson (1964)	–	–	–	–	50%	–
Townsend and Wedderburn (1965)	–	30%	–	–	–	–
Brockington and Lempert (1966)	–	–	–	–	54%	–
Goldberg (1970)	–	–	31%	–	–	–
Nottingham Social Services (1973)	–	–	–	32%	–	–
Milne (1976)	39%	–	44%	–	53%	–
Abrams (1978)	–	–	–	36%	–	–
Present study (self-estimate) 1980	–	–	38%	39%	54%	69%
Present study (based on audiometry) 1980	–	–	60%	69%	82%	84%

However, in keeping with all other studies where no audiometry was performed, only 38 per cent of the sample responded positively to the conventional question on the interview schedule regarding hearing loss. An analysis of studies which have assessed hearing loss on the judgement of the clinician or interviewer, have produced results equally at odds with the pure-tone audiometer (Gilhome Herbst 1982). Deafness is not easy to observe.

Incidence of dementia

Sixteen per cent of the sample were assessed as suffering from some degree of organic brain syndrome, a figure comparable with those of other studies reviewed by Gilmore (1974). As was to be expected, a significant relationship was found between increased age and incidence and severity of dementia (at the 0.1 per cent level).

Seventy-nine per cent of the demented were also deaf. Indeed as people get

TABLE 11.4. *Dementia by degree of deafness, controlled for age*

Age in years

Dementia	70 – 79				80 +			
	Degree of deafness				Degree of deafness			
	Not deaf 0–34 dB	Moderately and substantially deaf 35–69 dB	Severely deaf 70 dB+	Total	Not deaf 0–34 dB	Moderately and substantially deaf 35–69 dB	Severely deaf 70 dB+	Total
	No. (%)	No. (%)	No. (%)	No. (%)	No. (%)	No. (%)	No. (%)	No. (%)
Not demented	78 (94)	74 (88)	11 (85)	163 (91)	9 (75)	27 (66)	7 (58)	43 (66)
'Mild' and 'marked' dementia	5 (6)	10 (12)	2 (15)	17 (9)	3 (25)	14 (34)	5 (42)	22 (34)
Total	83 (100)	84 (100)	13 (100)	180 (100)	12 (100)	41 (100)	12 (100)	65 (100)

$\chi^2 = 2.27$ with 2 d.f.: not significant.

$\chi^2 = 0.75$ with 2 d.f.: not significant.

From Gilhome Herbst and Humphrey (1980), with permission.

deafer they are significantly more likely to be demented (at the 5 per cent level). However, our results do not support the suggestion made by Kay *et al*. 1964*b*) that the connection between deafness and dementia is 'too strong to be wholly explicable by advanced age'. Our work has shown that deafness is the norm for all elderly persons over the age of 80 years and once age was controlled for, the apparent relationship was lost (Table 11.4). Deafness and dementia appear to be merely contiguous conditions, but both are functions of age.

Incidence of depression

Thirty-five per cent of the sample were screened as depressed. These figures for depression are a little higher than other community studies (Kay *et al*. 1964*a*; Blessed 1979), but this may be explained by the slightly greater age of the respondents and the consequently higher proportion of women among whom the incidence of depression is apparently greater (Kay *et al*. 1964*b*). A significant relationship was found between age and depression (at the 5 per cent level) but there was no association between age and severity of depression.

Before we proceeded any further in our analysis of the association between deafness and depression in old age, we decided to withdraw the schedules of 19 respondents who were assessed as suffering from 'marked' dementia, on the grounds that their responses to the interview were judged to be unreliable. Our sample was thus reduced.

Deafness and depression

Sixty-nine per cent of the depressed were also deaf and a significant relationship was found between deafness of depression (at the 1 per cent level). However, no relationship could be found between severity of depression and severity of deafness. When age and socioeconomic status were controlled for (using ANOVA — an SPSS subprogram for analysis of variance), a significant relationship between deafness and depression remained (Table 11.5).

TABLE 11.5. *The relationship between depression and deafness*

Deafness	Depression Not depressed		'Limited' and 'pervasive' depression		Total	
	No.	(%)	No.	(%)	No.	(%)
Not deaf 0–34 dB	72	(50)	22	(31)	94	(43)
'Deaf' 35 dB+	73	(50)	50	(69)	123	(57)
Total	145	(100)	72	(100)	217	(100)

From Gilhome Herbst and Humphrey (1980), with permission.
$\chi^2 = 6.39$ with 1 d.f. $p < 0.01$.

The use of audiometric techniques of assessment has made it possible to establish that there is an association between deafness and depression which is not simply a function of differential reporting reflecting the emotional state of the respondent.

IMPLICATIONS

What are the implications of these findings? In the first place, the use of audiometric techniques to assess the prevalence of deafness in this study has disclosed almost double the estimates previously produced by other studies, all of which relied solely on patient self-report or clinical judgement. This gross discrepancy has been confirmed by the only two comparable studies where audiometry was used, both of which were concerned with the elderly in residential institutions (Burton 1976; Martin and Peckford 1978). Considerable doubt is cast, therefore, upon the validity of all studies concerned to establish presence of deafness, where no audiometry is carried out. Deafness must be seen as almost synonymous with aging and, as such, as a contributing factor to the social and psychological experience of nearly *all* old people.

In the second place, let us consider our so-called negative finding — that we could find no association between deafness and dementia. It is still possible that there is some link between dementia and deafness of early onset. However, as a strong component of dementia is poor memory recall, without recourse to longitudinal studies using audiometric techniques, no causal associations can be made. The lack of a causal link between these conditions does not alter the fact that they frequently co-exist in the same elderly person. This is important, given the increasingly current practice in both research and clinical contexts of using screening devices, in the form of standardized tests, to establish the presence of organic mental disorders. Indeed, our own measure, the CARE Schedule, is such a test.

Screening for dementia

In 1970 Irving *et al.* in their study investigating the 'Validity of some cognitive tests in the diagnosis of dementia', mentioned that tests had to be omitted because of defects of vision or hearing. Isaacs and Kennie (1973) made a similar point about the unsuitability of the 'Set Test' for rapid testing of mental functioning, for use with deaf subjects, and so on. In that 82 per cent of all those over 80 years and 89 per cent of the 'markedly' demented in this study were found to be deaf, the validity of all such screening devices would seem to be questionable.

However, by tackling the assessment and diagnosis procedures with the firm expectation that nearly all dements, and the majority of elderly depressives, are also deaf, it should be possible to overcome this problem. The experiences of the present team showed that severely deaf respondents were initially loathe to make the effort to respond to the interview schedule, until they realized that their communication difficulties were fully appreciated and would be allowed for. This often took a little time and its achievement was frequently rewarded by a noticeable improvement in the respondents' co-operation and interest and, therefore, performance.

I feel this raises questions about the positioning in interviews of screens for dementia, which require maximum concentration and yet are frequently placed too early on for good rapport to have been established between patient and clinician. It is essential to use great care, patience, and ingenuity, to ensure maximum audibility and visibility of the spoken word and to be prepared, if necessary, to use the written word (used by us quite frequently). I personally found that sitting on the floor, within easy and relaxed view of the elderly person, with the light firmly on my face helped enormously. In any event, conventional clinical techniques may prove inadequate, in which case there is a strong argument to suggest that no assumptions about mental state should be made without an audiogram.

Deafness and diagnosis

The danger of regarding, and therefore, treating, elderly people as demented or confused when they are actually severely deaf, is not hard to imagine, particularly as the manifestations of both these disorders are in many ways so similar. Such fears have already been voiced by researchers, particularly with regard to residents in local authority homes for the elderly (Townsend 1964; Martin and Peckford 1977).

Let us next consider our positive finding – namely the association of deafness with depression in the elderly living at home. For the sake of discussion, we proposed that elderly people living 'active' lives (much as they would have normally done during their middle years), were those who reported good health, did not describe themselves as lonely people, had no mobility problems and maintained an active relationship with friends as well as their families. These are the active elderly whom Isaacs would have considered in their 'silver' age (Isaacs 1974). Against these 'active' elderly, can be balanced the elderly living 'disengaged' lives. That is, those who reported living alone, had little or no supportive family network, no relationships with persons other than their family, no contacts outside the home, and had not left their homes during the last week.

Deafness interfered most with people at each of these extremes. For those with a way of life that might be more traditionally associated with the middle-aged, deafness was found to be as irksome as it is to people of younger years, and a stronger association between depression and deafness was found. At the other end of the spectrum, deafness was particularly bothersome for elderly people leading 'disengaged' lives. For such people, deafness increased their fears of personal insecurity and underlined the losses in their lives which had 'reduced them to this'. These people were also far more likely to feel lonely than any other group of elderly people and, most important, were most likely to be depressed. For the bulk of elderly people who live neither particularly active lives, nor particularly withdrawn lives, deafness seemed to matter far less. This explains, in part, the weak association (weaker than in those of employment age) of deafness with depression, and underlines the important role of life-style and life expectations in determining whether deafness is handicapping.

Scope for intervention

The scope for intervention is evidently wide, particularly amongst the 'young old'. Unfortunately, however, early diagnosis and treatment is substantially hampered by prevailing social attitudes to deafness, particularly amongst the elderly themselves but regretfully too by many general practitioners (Humphrey *et al.* 1981). Arguably this oversight is partly due to the insidious prevalence of deafness. At the present time there seems little evidence to suggest that not wearing a hearing aid actually worsens the *impairment*, that is the degree of deafness. However, without an aid the social and psychological effects of deafness, namely withdrawal, depression, and also the frustration of other people, are unalleviated and may feed back into the disorder, accentuating alienation and discrimination.

This study is unremarkable in its finding that only 13 per cent of the elderly population (of whom 60 per cent were 'deaf') possessed hearing aids, thus there is evidently vast scope for action. Whilst it may not be possible to say that deafness is a *major* cause of depression in old age, it is certainly a contributing factor and one which may be more readily ameliorated than many others. It might be pointed out that, with regard to the other common sensory defect in old age, namely failing sight, 97 per cent of the same sample possessed spectacles and this almost universal provision is taken for granted.

Acknowledgements

I should like to thank the Nuffield Foundation for funding the study and the Polytechnic of North London for its support. Thanks are due to the doctors of the general practice concerned, for granting access to their patients and to the receptionist at the practice, without whose generous help the study could not have been carried out. Much gratitude is also due to Ms Charlotte Humphrey for her invaluable support and to Ms J. Stevenson and Ms S. Faruqi, research assistants to the study, and to Dr E. Murphy who validated our administration of the CARE schedule.

REFERENCES

Abrams, M. (1978). *Beyond three-score and ten. A first report on a survey of the elderly*. Age Concern Research Publication, Mitcham.

Bergmann, K. (1977). Chronic brain failure — epidemiological aspects. *Age Ageing* 6, Suppl., 4-8.

Blessed, G. (1979). Depression: assessing the patient behind the mask. *Geriat. Med.* 29-32.

Brockington, F. and Lempert, S. M. (1966). *The social needs of the over-80s*. Manchester University Press.

Burton, D. K. (1976). Hearing impaired residents in local authority homes for the elderly. M. Sc. dissertation, Salford University.

Charatan, F. B. (1975). Depression in old age. *NY St. J. Med.* 75, 2505-7.

Cooper, A. F., Garside, R. F., and Kay, D. W. K. (1976). A comparison of deaf and non-deaf patients with paranoid and affective psychoses. *Br. J. Psychiat.* 129, 532-8.

Copeland, J. R. M., Kelleher, M. J., Kellett, J. M., Gourlay, A. J., Gurland, B. J., Fleiss, J. L., and Sharpe, L. (1976). A semi-structured clinical interview for the assessment of diagnosis and mental state in the elderly: the Geriatric Mental State Schedule. *Psychol. Med.* 6, 439-49.

Cosin, L. Z., Mort, M., Post, F., Westropp, C., and Williams, M. (1957). Persistent senile confusion: a study of 50 consecutive cases. *Int. J. Soc. Psychiat.* 3, 195-202.

Cumbria County Council (1973). *Survey of the handicapped and impaired and elderly over seventy-five in Cumberland*. Cumbria County Council.

Garland, M. H. (1978). Depression and dementia. *Hosp. Update* 313-19.

Gilhome Herbst, K. R. (1982). Some social implications of acquired deafness in ageing. In *Current trends in British gerontology* (ed. R. Taylor and A. Gilmore). Gower Press.

—— (1982). Psycho-social consequences of disorders of hearing in the elderly. In *Medicine in old age – hearing and balance* (ed. R. Hinchcliffe). Churchill Livingstone, Edinburgh.

—— and Humphrey, C. M. (1980). Hearing impairment and mental state in the elderly living at home. *Br. med. J.* **280**, 903-5.

—— —— (1981). Prevalence of hearing impairment in the elderly living at home. *J. R. Coll. gen. Pract.* **31**, 155-60.

Gilmore, A. J. J. (1974). Community surveys and mental health. In *Geriatric medicine* (ed. W. F. Anderson and T. G. Judge). Academic Press, London.

Goldberg, E. M. (1970). *Helping the aged.* National Institute of Social Work. Training Series 19. Allen and Unwin, London.

Gurland, B. J., Kuriansky, J. B., Sharpe, L., Simon, R., Stiller, P., and Birkett, P. (1977). The Comprehensive Assessment and Referral Evaluation (CARE) – rationale, development and reliability. *Int. J. Aging hum. Devl.* **8**, 9-42.

Harris, A. I. (1962). *The social survey. Health and welfare of older people in Lewisham.* Central Office of Information, London.

Harris, M., Thomas, A. J., and Lamont, M. (1981). Use of environmental aids by adults with severe sensorineural hearing loss – an exploratory study. *Br. J. Audiol.* **15**, 101-6.

Hodkinson, H. M. (1973). Mental impairment in the elderly. *J. R. Coll. Physicians* **7**, 305-17.

Humphrey, C. M., Gilhome Herbst, K. R., and Faruqi, S. (1981). Some characteristics of the hearing impaired elderly who do not present themselves for rehabilitation. *Br. J. Audiol.* **15**, 25-30.

Irving, G., Robinson, R. A., and McAdam, W. (1970). The validity of some cognitive tests in the diagnosis of dementia. *Br. J. Psychiat.* **117**, 149-56.

Isaacs, B. (1974). The silver age. *New Society* **30**, 417-18.

—— and Kennie, A. (1973). The Set Test as an aid to the detection of dementia in old people. *Br. J. Psychiat.* **123**, 467-70.

Kay, D. W. K., Beamish, P., and Roth, M. (1964a). Old age mental disorders in Newcastle upon Tyne. Part I: A study of prevalence. *Br. J. Psychiat.* **110**, 146-58.

—— —— —— (1964b). Old age mental disorders in Newcastle upon Tyne. Part II: A study of possible social and medical causes. *Br. J. Psychiat.* **110**, 668-82.

Martin, D. N. and Peckford, R. W. (1977). *Hearing impairment in homes for the elderly.* North Yorkshire County Council Social Services Department.

—— —— (1978). Hearing impairment in homes for the elderly. *Soc. Work Serv.* **17**, 52-62.

Milne, J. S. (1976). Hearing loss related to some signs and symptoms in older people. *Br. J. Audiol.* **10**, 65-73.

—— Maule, M. M., and Williamson, J. (1971). Method of sampling in a study of older people with a comparison of respondents and non-respondents. *Br. J. prevent. soc. Med.* **25**, 37-41.

Nottingham Social Services (1973). *The elderly in Nottingham. Report on phase I of a survey of persons aged 75+.* Nottingham Social Services Committee.

Post, F. (1958). Social factors in old age psychiatry. *Geriatrics* **13**, 567-80.

Richardson, I. M. (1964). *Age and need. A study of older people in the North-East of Scotland.* Livingstone, Edinburgh.

Sheard, A. V. (1971). Survey of the elderly in Scunthorpe. *Publ. Hlth, Lond.* **85**, 208-18.

Sheldon, J. H. (1948). *The social medicine of old age. Report of an enquiry in Wolverhampton.* Oxford University Press, London.

Thomas, A. J. and Gilhome Herbst, K. R. (1980*a*). Social and psychological implications of acquired hearing loss for adults of employment age. *Br. J. Audiol.* **14**, 76–85.

—— —— (1980*b*). Acquired deafness and psychological disorders. In *Disorders of auditory function*, Vol. III. *Proc. 3rd Conf. Br. Soc. Audiol.* (ed. I. G. Taylor) pp. 321–8. Academic Press, London.

—— and Ring, J. (1981). A validation of the Hearing Measurement Scale. *Br. J. Audiol.* **15**, 55–60.

Townsend, P. (1964). *The last refuge.* Routledge and Kegan Paul, London.

—— and Wedderburn, D. (1965). *The aged in the welfare state.* Occasional Papers on Social Administration, No. 14. Bell, London.

Wilkins, L. T. (1948). *The social survey. Survey of the prevalence of deafness in the population of England, Scotland and Wales.* Central Office of Information, London.

Williamson, J., Stokoe, I. H., Gray, S., Fisher, M., Smith, A., McGhee, A., and Stephenson, E. (1964). Old people at home: their unreported needs. *Lancet* i, 1117–20.

PART III
Psychiatric disorders

12

Anxiety in old age

ALEX COMFORT

It is not my experience that old age is a time of major anxiety, although one might well expect it to be, on realistic grounds. The old have to address many insecurities — social, financial, existential; they live with an ongoing process of bereavement, major and minor—loss of people, of roles, of skills, and of faculties, all of which call for mourning of greater or lesser degree. Mourning is not anxiety, but it contains the apprehension of further mourning to come. And yet, when one reviews a geropsychiatric population, anxiety is probably a less common complaint than it is in adolescence. Regret and disappointment are common, but so is a degree of acceptance or positive contentment.

That is not to say, of course, that anxiety does not figure in geriatric psychiatry — it does. In this context I do not want to deal with the area of realistic apprehension as, for example, the fear of becoming victims of crime among old folk in New York, or of being relegated to an American speculative nursing home. But we should not address these problems psychopharmacologically. The old in America, which is where I have been working with them, are frequent targets for minor tranquillizers, but so are younger adults. These drugs offer a convenient letout from addressing the problems of the society. The old run the additional risk, however, of getting major tranquillizers if they continue to complain, on the basis that they must be senile and need to be kept quiet at all costs.

INAPPROPRIATE USE OF TRANQUILLIZERS

The discussion of psychopharmacology in relation to geriatric anxiety might well begin here, because one common cause of the latter is medication. Folklore has long taught that, when one is old, one 'loses one's marbles', becomes 'gaga', or contracts 'senile dementia', presumably through no cause other than the passage of time.

Anxiety and dementia

One of the commonest anxieties in anxious old people is that this fate is beginning to overtake them. They may examine their mental processes rather as apprehensive males scrutinize their potency, and with similar results. The benign slowing of memory access with age reinforces their worries; Thomas Jefferson had the same anxiety when he found it hard to study mathematics as retentively as he had done in youth; it led him to reject the idea of a life Presidency. This anxiety may be covert, and only elicited when one gives reassurance, or it may be consuming. The liability to be anxious, after all, varies; chronic worriers and hypochondriacs remain chronic worriers and hypochondriacs when old. The important difference is that while minor tranquillizers and sedatives, or alcohol, may suppress anxiety of this kind in the young, in the old they aggravate it. For in the old, these drugs readily produce precisely the impairment of memory and orientation that the patient fears.

In true dementia of the Alzheimer type, anxiety about intellectual impairment is usually minor; it is the relatives who worry. Insight and consequent anxiety suggest a non-Alzheimer aetiology. For the non-demented person, serious mental impairment is intensely disturbing, and in a sizeable proportion of cases where anxiety over this is a presenting symptom, the patient is on benzodiazepines, tricyclic antidepressants, digoxin, uncompensated diuretics, or more than one of these. The intellectual impairment is genuine, and the treatment is to stop the medication, when it will recover. Bearing in mind that senility-phobia is commoner in the old than cancer-phobia, heart-disease-phobia and all the other health anxieties of the younger adult rolled into one, our first task in prescribing is to avoid inducing mental impairment due to the drugs administered. These include: sedatives, anticholinergic drugs, 'safe' hypnotics like flurazepam or nitrazepam which are major offenders in scrambling old folks' wits, and, in general, any powerful and unnecessary medication. It is a characteristic of the elderly population, that intellect is affected by drugs long before they grossly affect physiology elsewhere.

MANIFESTATIONS OF ANXIETY

Relocation panic

The commonest precipitant of isolated acute anxiety in the old is relocation; moving, that is, to another house or another town. The reasons for this are multiple and unfamiliarity is one of them. Most of us have experienced the unease called 'directional vertigo' when a tree is cut down or the garden fence is moved and in the old it is compounded, once again, by fear of senility. Particularly where, by misfortune, the new house or flat is a mirror image of the old one, moving can set off a severe anxiety attack. This can be dealt with by explanation, support, assisted re-learning of the new neighbourhood and brief sedation if the anxiety is extreme (and by brief I mean 12–24 hours, under close supervision). The drug which specifically suppresses unfamiliarity-anxiety in rats is propranolol, but a great many geriatric patients have conditions which contraindicate it, and it can of itself induce marked mental confusion in others (Kurland 1979). Eisdorfer, however, did show that in a healthy old population it improved test performance by lessening fear of failure (Eisdorfer *et al.* 1970), and there may be cases in our experience where it seems worth a careful trial.

One should regard relocational panic as a specific disorder, likening it to the panic states triggered in younger patients by heart-valve abnormalities. The mechanism, quite apart from 'soft ware' causes, such as sudden loss of previous social context and familiar objects, seems to depend on collision between the orientation reflex and the slower rate of adaption in old subjects. This explains why severe relocation panic can affect independent and hardheaded people, rather as it is said to affect Balinese islanders removed from Bali.

Placid hypochondriasis

I have dealt at length with relocation panic, because, apart from it, panic states in the old are rather rare. One may see them in multiembolic dementia, the so-called 'catastrophic crisis'. One may also see neurotics grown old in neurosis, for neurosis is not, it seems, aggravated by age (Bergmann 1978). Nor does it become commoner, but anxious hyperreaction to the particular stresses imposed by society on the old, takes the place of what we may call 'young' anxieties (Ernst 1959), which need a larger sense of futurity to have scope. Anxiety over death is an adolescent preoccupation, not a geriatric one. The commonest manifestation of neurosis in the old is angry or apprehensive, but placid hypochondriasis, in which the patient seems to be trying to communicate, or unload, his anxiety on the physician. I do not propose to discuss the management of hypochondriasis; suffice it to say that the day centre plays an important role, since the hypochondriac is often the resident host or hostess there, encouraging others to somatize.

Unrecognized depression

There is a pharmacologically critical differential diagnosis between hypochondriasis and the commonest cause of non-episodic, unprecipitated major anxiety in old age, namely unrecognized depression. Hypochondriacs do not commit suicide: depressed patients do. It pays to remember, faced with a sudden, non-relocational access of anxiety in a previously robust old patient, that first unipolar depressive attacks do not become less frequent until the eighth decade (Post 1968). When they are mild and agitation prevails over depressed affect, they are commonly missed.

Now that we have effective antidepressants it is important to stress the depression of old age, which affects some 15 per cent of persons over 70, and which is a diagnostic before it becomes a therapeutic problem. Both the old and their doctors tend to expect dysphoria in age and miss its causes because, in these cases, the degree of masked depression can be judged only when it is lifted. Patients which are frankly depressed are fortunate, for we do not miss them. Those we miss present with anergia, dysphoria, anxiety, or a mixture of these. We also attribute hypochondriasis to the old, who have realistic reasons to be apprehensive about their health, and who are lonely and like to visit the doctor. I think that the best diagnostic distinction here lies in the fact that the depressed subject blames himself, while the hypochondriac blames you, your predecessors, and medicine generally. No hypochondriac believes that his illness is terminal but depressed people often do. Hypochondriacs tend to sleep and eat well, to have histories of health worries but not of mood changes, and to retain their weight. And hypochondriacs do not commit suicide. It is a definite danger sign when an older patient commenses *uncharacteristic* return visits, and displays *uncharacteristic* anxiety mixed with resignation which inquiry shows to be a cover for despair.

TREATMENT IN THE ELDERLY
Treatment always tends to be a little out-of-date. We have been seeing patients in a correctly diagnosed anxious depression who have been routinely put on full doses of amitriptyline. The message we probably need to convey is that old

people tend to do rather badly on tricyclics. They experience severer side-effects, blood levels tend to swing unpredictably, and, in particular, anticholinergic drugs exacerbate anxiety by causing confusion and memory loss. The non-anticholinergic or less anticholinergic drugs such as desipramine, can be anxiogenic and produce akathisia in the old.

The role of MAOI

Since I began working in America I have seen a striking move in geriatric practice away from tricyclics, even in low doses − 25 mg of doxepin instead of 75 mg or more per day −towards tetracyclics, which are still experimental but seem promising, and still more towards monamine oxidase inhibitors (MAOI), phenelzine in particular. American physicians have been terrified of MAOIs, and a number of texts and lectures have described them as unsuitable for geriatric use; partly on the ground that the old will not adhere to a diet, and partly for fear of their interaction with emergency medication. These fears are apparently quite misplaced. Phenelzine has the advantage for old patients of being specifically antiphobic, not having disturbing or hazardous cardiac and anticholinergic side-effects, and working best on the 'atypical' depressions, those with anergia plus anxiety, which are most often missed in the old. When it has to be stopped, this is usually because of hypotension, not hypertensive crisis. Since so much *de novo* anxiety at geriatric ages is depressive in origin, MAOIs seem to have a major place in its treatment. They also have the great advantage, where they do act, of acting rapidly. I think the management of anxiety in old age, where it calls for drugs, now centres on amoxapine, phenelzine, and occasionally doxepin, not chlordiazepoxide, which has taken the place of phenobarbitone. Still less, as some advertisers and nursing-home aides seem to want us to believe, is haloperidol ever indicated.

Psychiatrically the interaction of realistic apprehension, chronic anxiety-proneness, mourning, and genuine late-life depression is pretty difficult to unravel, especially when history-taking is complicated by deafness, but it needs to be done, and done thoroughly. My feeling from reviewing cases is that if we can exclude relocation anxiety, longstanding and unremitting worry-proneness which is part of a long-established style, factors in the real environment which would make any reasonable person apprehensive, and misinformation about the normal course of aging, and when we have reassured the patient that major illness and incipient dementia are not present and have reviewed all medications, we should adopt a variant of Lewis and Piotrowski's notorious dictum (1954) that 'any trace of schizophrenia is schizophrenia' and assume that any trace of affective disorder in the old is affective disorder. The second dictum is correct − the first isn't.

Recognizing anxiety

One does often have a serious diagnostic problem in drawing a distinction between anxiety, which occurs with an intact sensorium and brain, and agitation, which accompanies dementia or brain damage. Post-stroke patients can have either, or more usually both. Agitation does indeed respond to miniscule doses of haloperidol, but the risk is that any state of restlessness or apprehension in the old will be taken for an incurable part of the dementing process, while in fact we may be seeing anxiety. Anxiety at being in a nursing home (a very reasonable frame of mind, judging from some American nursing homes), at some extramural activity of relatives or their failure to visit, over how a spouse is faring—or even quite simply over being divorced from a favourite TV programme. An old lady who every night quartered the hospital muttering, was labelled 'demented', until someone took the trouble to listen to what she muttered. It was 'Johnny Carson, Johnny Carson'. Provision of a television set worked in this case where haloperidol did not. In others it will be simply a matter of the patience to penetrate sensory barriers and find out what is on the patient's mind. In the minority of cases which do need sedation, as for example when a spouse is dying or surgery is imminent, oxazepam seems to do least harm (Steinhart 1978) because it does not tend to accumulate long-term metabolites. But it is not a substitute for communication with the patient. One can assess the psychiatric trouble taken in a ward of assorted seniors, by noting the number and frequency of prescriptions as designated by: o.n. or h.s. or t.d.s. and not p.r.n., in the Cardex file.

Sleep, and anxiety about it, would merit an entire book. The depressed insomniac with early waking may put down his dysphoria to the bad nights he has, and focus anxiety on it. Anxious old people who are not depressed are targets for hypnotics, worse insomnia, and iatrogenic anxiety about their lack of sleep. During drug withdrawal the most effective medication is hot milk, self-selection of hours of sleep and waking, and sufficient human company to induce tranquillity of mind. On the rare occasion when a hypnotic is given for the benefit of the patient, rather than the staff who are in bad conscience and have been led to share the patient's concern, I agree with Stotsky in the unfashionable choice of a minute dose of butobarbitone over more fashionable and widely-promoted medications (Stotsky *et al*. 1971). In my view there are no indications for any hypnotic o.n. When many of these are being ordered, the institution is due for what the Russians call 'self-criticism', directed to the patients' quality of life.

CAUSES OF ANXIETY IN THE ELDERLY

I want to revert, finally, to the part that the image of decrepit and demented old age plays in making the old anxious. We are all apprehensive when we visit a doctor for if we had no concerns we would not be seeing him. But this squeam-ishness is readily aggravated even in the most robust senior, by the reception he gets in the receiving room or from the receptionist, or from the doctor himself. I tell Americans that every old patient feels in the waiting-room a little like a Jew who thinks that the staff may possibly be Nazis, or a Black who thinks they may be racists. Address him as 'dad', or ask him if he knows his name and what day of the week it is, and you have an anxious as well as an angry patient ready-made. Even routine mental tests can arouse intense apprehension. I like to think that in England the devaluation of oldness has not gone so far. It is the physician, insensitive to the verbal and non-verbal cues his practice is giving out to geriatric patients, who leans most heavily on sedatives, tranquillizers, and antipsychotics.

One answer to overmedication may be more geriatricians; another is more old doctors. Unfortunately it is the insensitive and scientoid whom psychopharmacology today provides with live ammunition and active placebos.

I very much regret the passing of that invaluable therapeutic aid to minor psychiatry, the bottle of medicine. It was the ideal transitional object, embodying the physician's concern in a form visible to relatives; it had no side-effects, it could not be diverted to suicide and it was as effective therapeutically in many contexts as the active medications which have replaced it. I will hope that one day this society may convene a meeting on the subject 'How can we replace the bottle of medicine?'; In one respect it aided the physician; by requiring repeated visits for refilling it gave time to assess the most important indicator in geriatric psychiatry and geriatric medicine, namely change. Usually in hospital we are forced to assess patients who have no family doctor (under the American system he is replaced by a self-selected host of non-communicating specialists) and whom we have never seen before. The geriatric psychiatrist in Britain is more fortunate, since he is more likely to have access to the patient's track record. Having this, anxiety which arises suddenly in the old can be recognized and its causes identified; chronic anxiety can be addressed by a form of psychotherapy to which the old alone have access, namely the use of reminiscence. This being done, it is not too late to undertake psychotherapy in a form apt to the older patient.

REFERENCES

Bergmann, K. (1978). In *Studies in geriatric psychiatry* (ed. A. D. Isaacs and F. Post). Wiley, New York.
Eisdorfer, C., Nowlin, J., and Wilkie, F. (1970). *Science, NY* **170**, 1327.
Ernst, K. (1959). *Monogr. Neurol. Psychiat.* **85**.
Kurland, M. L. (1979). *New Engl. J. Med.* **300**, 366.
Lewis, N. D. C. and Piotrowski, Z. A. (1954). In *Depression* (ed. P. Hock and J. Zubin). Grune and Stratton, New York.
Post, F. (1968). In *Studies in geriatric psychiatry* (ed. A. D. Isaacs and F. Post). Wiley, New York.
Steinhart, M. J. (1978). *Consultant* **18**, 137.
Stotsky, B., Cole, J. O., and Yang, Y. T. (1971). *J. Am. geriat. Soc.* **19**, 860.

13

Treatment of depression in old age

STUART A. MONTGOMERY

In all developed countries the aged have increased in absolute numbers and are increasing as a proportion of the population. Indeed the fastest rate of growth has been seen in the over 75 year age group, and in the United Kingdom this rate of increase is not expected to change much before the end of the century. The problem of provision of care for this growing elderly population is a matter of concern for the immediate future, and is exacerbated by the concurrent decline in the size of the economically active population. The elderly are major users of health services, occupying half the medical beds and nearly half the psychiatric beds, in hospitals in the United Kingdom.

The elderly have a high incidence of both mental and physical illness, much of which is irremediable. However, the careful diagnosis of psychiatric illness that is treatable, will improve the quality of life of the old person, as well as doing much to reduce the burden on agencies concerned with the management of the elderly. There is currently recognition of the fact that psychiatric care for the elderly has been underprovided. To some extent this stems from a still quite prevalent attitude of resignation which regards old age as a time of inevitable decline, incapacity, and gloom. The pessimism and apathy so frequently seen in old people are taken to be a normal consequence of aging, but such despondency may, and frequently does, represent an undetected treatable depressive illness. Estimates of the prevalence of depressive illness in the elderly vary quite widely and it is probable that depressive illness is one of the most frequent untreated psychiatric disorders in this group. A recent study (Busse 1978) showed that in a sample of 209 people in the community over the age of 65, 20 per cent reported significant depressive episodes during the past three years. Other incidence studies have put the figure higher still.

PROBLEMS OF DIAGNOSIS

Much treatable depression may be missed by the clinician because of the complicated clinical picture presented by the elderly. Diagnosis of depression in the aged is confounded by a number of factors. External factors certainly play a part in determining apparent psychopathology in behaviour patterns. Loss of interest in previously pleasurable activities may be a response to naturally dwindling energy levels. Eating patterns may be affected even in an active elderly person who finds himself in social isolation to which he has not been accustomed.

Medical illness

This is far more prevalent in the older age group and may mask or mimic depressive symptomatology. Some physical illness, for example neoplasia, may manifest itself in the early stages with behavioural changes. Metabolic disturbances such as abnormalities of serum glucose, potassium, calcium, and hepatic dysfunction; endocrine disturbances such as hypothyroidism; and infectious diseases, can all lead to apathy, lack of activity and anorexia. These physical disorders may initially present clinically as depression. Such symptoms are more difficult to assess in the elderly than in younger patients, because the variation between elderly individuals in level of normal functioning is very much wider.

Concurrent medication

Another factor is that old people are more likely to be taking medication for other ailments. It has been established that the number of medicines a patient is prescribed increases with age (Parry *et al.* 1973). The regimens of elderly patients with multiple problems can reach formidable proportions, and there is a risk of polypharmacy escalating benign elderly forgetfulness into confusion, with resultant loss of strict compliance. There is the added complication that some drugs which are prescribed more frequently for the elderly can produce the symptoms of depression. Hypertension is one of the disorders that increases with age so that more elderly people are treated with antihypertensives some of which, e.g. guanethidine, and methyldopa, can cause apparent depression. Other classes of drugs such as some of the antianxiety drugs, hypnotics and corticosteroids, can have a similar effect. The possibility of such physical causes of symptomatology must be eliminated before embarking on antidepressant therapy.

Hypochondriasis

Depression in the elderly tends to manifest itself with somatic symptoms, and the patient frequently complains of specific or non-specific pains, discomforts, or general unwellness. One could speculate that this serves an adaptive function in bringing the patient to medical attention which might otherwise be denied. The attitude that old age is primarily a time of regret, disappointment, and loss, and the cultural norm that adversity is to be borne with fortitude, may well cause the elderly depressed patient to focus his disorder on physical symptoms. This preoccupation with somatic symptoms can reach hypochondriacal levels. Because the presenting complaints are so frequently somatic and the risk of physical disorder is high in the elderly, it is not surprising that physical causes are sought. There may sometimes be considerable delay before the patient's illness is recognized as having a psychological basis.

Pseudodementia

As has been emphasized in the previous chapter, much depression in the elderly is also probably overlooked, because of a bias towards the diagnosis of dementia. Confusion and memory impairment are common features of many illnesses in old people including depression. There is a comparative paucity of clear criteria for the diagnosis of dementia, and the cognitive disability seen with depression may easily be misdiagnosed .as dementia. In many of these patients if the depression is treated the 'dementia' also disappears.

In general where there is a classic persistent endogenous depression, with guilt, sleep disturbance, diurnal swing, etc., the condition will not be misdiagnosed. Where, however, there is a history of recent bereavement or loss, the psychopathology of treatable depression may be easily overlooked and attributed too readily to understandable sadness occurring in the circumstances.

RESPONSE TO ANTIDEPRESSANTS

Our knowledge about the efficacy of antidepressants in the treatment of depression in the elderly, has been to some extent restricted by the apparent exclusion of elderly patients from clinical trials of comparative antidepressant effect. The difficulty of making the primary diagnosis of depressive illness in the elderly may be one reason for this exclusion. In some research units there is already a selection factor operating, as there is a tendency for the aged not to be admitted to psychiatric units. Physical infirmity may confuse the assessment of severity of depression, whilst cognitive impairment will certainly make the use of self-rating questionnaires difficult or impossible in some patients. It is hardly surprising that there have been so few well-controlled studies of antidepressant efficacy using careful trial methodology, in the elderly.

Opinion is divided as to whether the elderly respond less well to antidepressant pharmacotherapy than younger patients. Patients who have suffered from episodes of depression early in life are likely to suffer from further episodes in late life, although if they have responded to antidepressant drugs in the past they are likely to do so again.

Older and younger compared

To establish if there is a difference in overall response between older and younger patients we have compared the response of a series of 186 patients suffering from depression, on the basis of a division by age at 55 years. Previous findings have indicated that other differences, such as differences in pharmacokinetics, may be observed between patients above and below this age (Montgomery *et al.* 1978*a*).

The patients were all participating in controlled double-blind trials and were being treated with an antidepressant (following a placebo washout period to reduce placebo responders). The group aged 55 years and over had a significantly poorer reponse, as measured by the final Hamilton Rating Scale (HRS) score, than the younger age group ($z = 2.47, p < 0.01$). The younger group were divided into further age cohorts but no significant difference in response was seen. When the older age group was divided into those aged 65 years and over and those below 65, the older age group had a slightly better outcome, though not significantly so. The contention that the elderly do not respond as well to pharmacotherapy was not confirmed in our analysis.

The explanation for this difference in response is probably multifactorial. Qualitative differences in the depression and biochemical factors relating to treatment may play a part. The search for secure predictors of response remains a major concern, in order to treat appropriate patients with relevant antidepressants.

168   Treatment of depression in old age

A review of studies of tricyclic antidepressant efficacy has suggested there are some common factors such as, for example, insidious onset, reduced sleep and appetite, that are associated with better response (Bielski and Friedel 1976). However, there are considerable methodological problems with such comparisons.

Endogenous and non-endogenous depression

With imipramine, antidepressant efficacy has been demonstrated most clearly in endogenous depression (Rogers and Clay 1975). The presence of life events on their own is insufficient for the diagnosis of non-endogenous depression. In the older age group for example, a higher incidence of stressful loss events may lead to the overdiagnosis of reactive depression, and treatable endogenous depression may be overlooked. The Newcastle Inventories (Carney et al. 1965; Gurney et al. 1972) may be used to categorize patients as suffering from endogenous depression where biological factors are more apparent, and non-endogenous depression where personality and environmental factors appear to have more influence.

In our series of depressed patients Newcastle Inventories were completed for 138 patients. We found that there was a trend for the proportion of endogenous depression to be greater in the over 55-year-old group than in those under 55 years. There is some evidence (Rama Rao and Coppen 1979) that patients with a high score on the reactive endogenous continuum, as measured by the Newcastle Inventory, have a poorer outcome to their illness, as measured by the final HRS score, than those in the mid-range. This might be of interest in the light of our finding of an association of a poorer outcome in the group aged over 55.

The usefulness of the endogenous reactive categorization for the prediction of response to different antidepressant drugs has still not been entirely elucidated. An unequivocal demonstration of antidepressant efficacy of imipramine was less likely in mixed or undifferentiated groups, but this might simply reflect the use of less careful methodology. Certainly there are studies which have found the response of both categories to be of a similar order, at least with some antidepressants. For example, mianserin has been found to be equally effective in endogenous and non-endogenous depression (Montgomery et al. 1978b), although a plasma level response relationship was seen only in the endogenous group.

There is a lack of well-controlled clinical investigations into the relative response of elderly depressed patients to specific antidepressants. Pharmacokinetic factors and consideration of safety and acceptability must, however, influence the choice of treatment.

Pharmacokinetic factors

As has been described in Chapter 5, the process of aging affects many factors influencing the disposition of drugs. Drug pharmacokinetics and dynamics may be affected by the changes seen with aging in the ratio of adipose tissue to protein in the body, in the total body water, in renal and liver function, and in receptor-site activity.

Because of the wide interindividual variation in the plasma levels of tricyclic antidepressants (TCAs) seen in patients receiving the same dose, the difference in response seen at different plasma levels is important. The findings are most consistent with nortriptyline, with which high drug plasma levels have been shown to be associated with poorer outcome. The same kind of effect is seen in studies of amitriptyline which is metabolized to nortriptyline. There are also a growing number of reports of an association between age and high plasma levels of anti-depressants. It is possible, as first reported in a study of the plasma concentration and clinical response relationship of mianserin (Montgomery *et al.* 1978*a*), that a correlation between drug plasma levels and age may be obscured by the phenomen of increased interindividual variability of plasma levels seen with age.

Age and plasma levels

In our group significant correlations have been reported between age and plasma concentrations, in studies on mianserin (Montgomery *et al.* 1978*a*), nortriptyline (Montgomery *et al.* 1980), zimelidine and norzimelidine (Montgomery *et al.* 1981). There is also evidence of some increased variability of levels with age with most antidepressants.

It is generally accepted by clinicians that the elderly require a lower dose than younger patients. The increased variability of plasma concentrations with age, and the deleterious effect of high levels seen for example with amitriptyline and nortriptyline, support this clinical view.

The benefit to be gained from possible improvement in clinical efficacy would be a sufficient reason for monitoring a patient's plasma concentrations. This is a time-consuming procedure and can entail a patient remaining on an inappropriate dosage, while steady state concentrations are being reached. However, single-dose pharmacokinetic tests have been devised for the prediction of steady state plasma concentrations (Montgomery *et al.* 1979). Dosage can be tailored for the individual patient on the basis of this test before treatment is begun.

TRICYCLIC CARDIOTOXICITY

There is evidence that some side-effects are also related to plasma concentrations. It is frequently noted that older depressed patients appear to suffer more severely from side-effects of antidepressants than younger patients. Subjectively experienced side-effects have not however been shown to be consistently correlated with plasma concentrations, despite occasional reports to the contrary.

Side-effects experienced by the patients may lead to treatment failure because of non-compliance. However, cardiotoxic effects of some TCAs which appear to be related to drug plasma concentrations would seem more dangerous. In view of their pharmacological actions it would be expected that the TCAs would have an effect on the cardiovascular system. Non-specific ST-T segment changes on the ECG were first reported in depressed patients being treated with imipramine following exercise (Kristiansen 1961). Various abnormalities have been reported since then for other TCAs as well as imipramine, and these include sinus tachy-cardia, conduction defects, ST-T wave abnormalities, ventricular arrhythmias, bradycardia, and asystole.

Risk of cardiotoxicity is associated with the TCAs not only in overdosage but also in therapeutic dosage. Amitriptyline has been implicated as a cause of sudden death in depressed patients receiving routine treatment for depression

(Coull *et al.* 1970). There have been an increasing number of investigations into the relative effects on the cardiovascular system of different antidepressants and it is a consistent finding that there are conduction disturbances and decreased contractility with the traditional TCAs (Burgess *et al.* 1979; Burrows *et al.* 1976).

It has been demonstrated, both in overdosage and in therapeutic dosage, that cardiotoxicity is related to plasma concentrations of TCA (Spiker *et al.* 1975; Taylor and Braithwaite 1978; Fensbo 1976). Treatment of the elderly with these traditional TCAs is more risky because of the increased variability of plasma levels reported. The same dose which produces therapeutic levels in one patient may produce potentially toxic levels in another. There is a higher incidence of cardiac disease in the elderly, but routine ECG screening before instituting treatment with TCAs is unfortunately not adequate in identifying the vulnerable patient. As with all difficult clinical decisions the risks associated with treatment have to be weighed against the risk of the illness, and the clinician must be aware that depression is life endangering.

Alternative antidepressants

Because of the risks associated with the TCAs in the elderly it has been suggested that alternative antidepressants are used. There is dissatisfaction with the traditional TCAs for patients of any age because of the associated cardiotoxicity, unacceptable side-effects and because they are only effective in two-thirds of patients. These problems are of greater significance in the elderly than in younger patients. The side-effects of TCAs can be experienced as so unpleasant as to interfere with treatment in all age groups, but some effects may have more serious consequences for the elderly. For example, postural hypotension which may be experienced as discomfort by a young physically healthy patient, may lead to falls and fractures in an elderly patient. Effects on cardiac contractility may not cause disability in the young and healthy, but in the elderly they could lead to cardiac failure, confusional states, and more serious complications.

The newer antidepressants have been developed in response to the need for safer and more acceptable antidepressants. The antidepressant action of some of these was discovered by chance, whilst others are the result of a systematic search for compounds which, because they have more selective actions, might have less unwanted effects. Results from studies on the possible cardiotoxic effects of the newer antidepressants compared with the TCAs appear to be favourable to the newer drugs. Mianserin, nomifensine, and zimelidine all appear to have less effect in therapeutic dosage on cardiac function than the reference TCAs (Burgess *et al.* 1979; Montgomery and Taylor 1980). It could therefore be expected that they would also be safer in overdosage than the TCAs. While it is still too early for adequate data to have been collected for zimelidine, both mianserin and nomifensine have been reported to be relatively safe in overdosage. In view of the risk of suicide associated with depression, which increases with age, this safety aspect of the newer antidepressants is important.

The acceptability of the newer compounds also appears to be an improvement although some side-effects are reported. Mianserin, for example, causes drowsiness and zimelidine loss of appetite. However, in comparisons with reference TCAs the level of side-effects has been reported to be significantly less with the new antidepressants (Coppen *et al.* 1976; Montgomery *et al.* 1981). If the newer antidepressants are as efficacious as the traditional TCAs, the findings of relative safety and acceptability would constitute strong arguments in favour of their use in the treatment of the elderly.

FUTURE APPROACHES

Further understanding of the psychopathological processes involved in depression in the elderly may be gained from some of the more recent approaches to the study of dementia. There is a suggestion that dementia may be linked with disturbances of specific metabolic pathways and the successful treatment of Parkinsonism with L-dopa has encouraged this view. The possibility that L-dopa might be effective in treating dementia has not been substantiated. However, an alternative approach is to investigate the use of some of the newer antidepressants which have a selective effect on 5HT metabolism. This is an interesting possibility, as 5HT is known to play a part in the regulation of dopamine metabolism. A link in some cases between dementia and depression in the elderly is an interesting hypothesis, and investigaton is welcomed in this area, which is likely to contribute to our knowledge of the processes affecting depression.

REFERENCES

Bielski, R. J. and Friedel, R. O. (1976). Prediction of antidepressant responses. *Archs gen. Psychiat.* **33**, 1479–89.
Burgess, C. D., Montgomery, S. A., Turner, P., and Wadsworth, J. (1979). Cardiovascular effects of amitriptyline, mianserin, zimelidine and nomifensine in depressed patients. *Postgrad. med. J.* **55**, 704–8.
Burrows, G. D., Vohra, J., Hunt, D., Sloman, J. G., Scoggins, B. A., and Davis, B. (1976). Cardiac effects of different tricyclic antidepressant drugs. *Br. J. Psychiat.* **129**, 335–41.
Busse, F. W. (1978). The Duke longitudinal study: I Senescence and senility. In *Alzheimer's disease; senile dementia and related disorders* (ed. R. Katzman, R. Terry, and K. Bick). Raven Press, New York.
Carney, M. W. P., Roth, M., and Garside, R. F. (1965). The diagnosis of depressive syndromes and the prediction of ECT response. *Br. J. Psychiat.* **111**, 659–4.
Coppen, A., Gupta, R., Montgomery, S., Ghose, K., Bailey, J., and de Ridder, J. J. (1976). Mianserin hydrochloride: a nodel antidepressant. *Br. J. Psychiat.* **129**, 342–5.
Coull, D. C., Crooks, J., Dingwall-Fordyce, I., Scott, A., and Weir, R. D. (1970). Amitriptyline and cardiac disease. Risk of sudden death identified by monitoring system. *Lancet* ii, 590.
Fensbo, D. (1976). A clinical trial of nortriptyline and maprotiline with cardiovascular monitoring and serum level estimations. Ludiomil Symposium, Malta.
Gurney, C., Roth, M., Garside, R. F., Kerr, T. A., and Shapira, K. (1972). Studies in the classification of affective disorders. *Br. J. Psychiat.* **121**, 162–6.
Kristiansen, E. S. (1961). Cardiac complications during treatment with imipramine (Tofranil). *Acta psychiat. neurol.* **36**, 427–42.
Montgomery, S. A., McAuley, R., and Montgomery, D. B. (1978a). The relationship between mianserin plasma levels and antidepressant effect in a double blind trial comparing a single night time and divided daily dose regimens.

Br. J. clin. Pharmac. **5**, 77S–80S.
— — — Braithwaite, R. A., and Dawling, S. (1979). Dosage adjustment from simple nortriptyline spot level predictor tests in depressed patients. *Clin. Pharmacokin.* **4**, 129.
— — — Dawling, S., and Braithwaite, R. A. (1980). Pharmacokinetics and efficacy of maprotiline and amitriptyline in endogenous depression. A double blind controlled trial. *Clin. Ther.* **3**, 292–310.
— — Rani, S. J., Roy, D., and Montgomery, D. B. (1981). A double blind comparison of zimelidine and amitriptyline in endogenous depression. *Acta psychiat. scand.* **63**, Suppl. 290, 314–27.
— Montgomery, D. B;. McAuley, R., and Rani, S. J. (1978*b*). Mianserin plasma levels and differential clinical response in endogenous and reactive depression. *Acta psychiat. belg.* **78**, 798–812.
— and Taylor, D. J. E. (1980). Cardiac effect of nomifensine, imipramine and amitriptyline in depressed patients. *R. Soc. Med. Symp.* **25**, 23–5.
Parry, J. J., Balter, M. B., and Mellinger, G. D. (1973). National patterns of psychotherapeutic drug use. *Archs gen. Psychiat.* **28**, 769.
Rama Rao, V. A. and Coppen, A. (1979). Classification of depression and response to amitriptyline therapy. *Psychol. Med.* **9**, 321–5.
Rogers, S. C. and Clay, P. M. (1975). A statistical review of controlled trials of imipramine and placebo in the treatment of depressive illness. *Br. J. Psychiat.* **127**, 599.
Spiker, D. G., Weiss, A. N., Chang, S. S., Ruwitch, J. F., and Biggs, J. T. (1975). Tricyclic antidepressant overdose: clinical presentation and plasma levels. *Clin. Pharmac. Ther.* **18**, 539–46.
Taylor, D. J. E. and Braithwaite, R. A. (1978). Cardiac effects of tricyclic antidepressant medication. A preliminary study of nortriptyline. *Br. Heart J.* **40**, 1005–9.

14

Treatment of sleep disturbance in the elderly

P. W. OVERSTALL

The first question to ask before prescribing a hypnotic for an old person is not 'Which one should I choose?' but 'Should I prescribe one at all?'. The risk of adverse reactions and addiction, and the doubtful long-term efficacy of many hypnotics, should make one cautious when responding to a patient who complains of insomnia.

The elderly receive more hypnotics than other age groups, and by the eighth decade 45 per cent are taking them regularly (McGhie and Russell 1962). Consumption is mainly by women, and they are more likely to complain of disturbed sleep than men, although analysis of electroencephalogram (EEG) recordings shows that at nearly all ages, men awaken more often than women (Williams et al. 1974). Personality is an important factor in determining whether a person will complain of insomnia; extroverts sleep for longer than introverts (Costello and Smith 1963) and also rate their sleep quality as significantly improved after receiving a hypnotic, whereas introverts do not (Oswald et al. 1975).

There is also the matter of expectation. Sleep patterns change with increasing age, and even healthy old persons should not expect to sleep as well as they did when young. The old person has reduced deep slow-wave sleep (stage 4), wakes more frequently, and has a longer sleep latency (the time taken to fall asleep). Pain, anxiety, and depression are particularly common causes of insomnia in the elderly, and they need appropriate treatment rather than a hypnotic. Unless care is taken in selecting patients who are likely to benefit from a hypnotic and in carefully reviewing them at frequent intervals, about one-third will still be taking the hypnotic one year later (Clift 1972). Moreover these patients rate the quality of their sleep as worse than those not on hypnotics (Gerard et al. 1978), which raises doubts as to the benefits of these drugs in the long term.

CHOOSING A HYPNOTIC

Most hypnotics are effective for one to three nights, but with repeated use, many have lost their effectiveness after one or two weeks (Kales and Kales 1975). Hypnotic trials in the elderly have recently been reviewed by Mendelson (1980) who concluded that no hypnotic has been shown to be particularly advantageous. Chronic hypnotic users have as great or greater difficulty in falling asleep or staying asleep, or both, as insomniac controls not taking drugs. The drugs are not merely inactive, for the chronic users have EEG changes, particularly a decrease in REM (rapid eye movement) sleep. Ideally, hypnotics should be used for short periods when it is clear that insomnia is impairing the patient's daytime performance. When choosing, the ensuing points should be considered.

Onset of action

It is essential that the drug should act rapidly if the patient's main complaint is difficulty in falling asleep. Many of the commonly-used hypnotics have a rapid rate of absorption (depending on the formulation) resulting in high and early peak concentrations. For example, peak plasma concentration occurs within 30 min of an oral dose of chlormethiazole (Briggs *et al*. 1980), in 60 min after temazepam (Fuccella 1979) and, on average, after 80 min with nitrazepam (Breimer *et al*. 1977). Two benzodiazepines which are unsuitable as hypnotics are oxazepam and lorazepam, since peak plasma concentrations are not reached for 2–2.5 h (Curry and Whelpton 1979).

Production of normal sleep

This used to be considered important, and the barbiturates were criticized because of their disruptive effect on EEG patterns. However, all hypnotics appear to cause some changes in sleep stages, and the significance of this is unknown. All that can be said of clinical relevance, is that abrupt withdrawal of a hypnotic which suppresses REM sleep, is often followed by a rebound effect associated with increased frequency of dreams and nightmares (Kales *et al*. 1974).

Hangover

This is of vital concern to the elderly, particularly those who are physically and mentally frail. Adverse effects are largely due to the accumulation of long-acting drugs and their metabolites, although there may also be an age-related increased sensitivity to the drug. The amount of accumulation is closely related to the plasma elimination half-life of the drug and its metabolites. A drug given once a day will inevitably accumulate if the elimination half-life exceeds 16.6 hours (Wagner 1967).

All the barbiturates used as hypnotics (with the exception of hexobarbital) have very long half-lives. Prolonged administration to elderly patients reverses sleep rhythm causing drowsiness by day, but confusion, restlessmess, and even excitement at night (Howell 1960; Gibson 1966). A pseudodementia may result, characterized by drowsiness, apathy, blunting of all the faculties, and a tendency to fall (Rudd 1972). The problem of falls has been highlighted by a report showing that over 90 per cent of elderly patients with a femoral fracture from a nocturnal fall, had been taking barbiturates (Macdonald and Macdonald 1977), although a similar survey by Brocklehurst *et al*. (1977) produced much less dramatic figures.

The long-acting benzodiazepines may also produce unwanted hangover effects in the form of daytime drowsiness, blurring of vision, and unsteadiness. The problems caused by nitrazepam in the elderly were first pointed out by Evans and Jarvis (1972), who described a characteristic syndrome of confusion, disorientation, dysarthria, incontinence, and falls. These symptoms can occur with as little as 5 mg a night and in patients who have been taking nitrazepam without ill-effect for some time.

In healthy old persons the pharmacokinetics of nitrazepam are unchanged (plasma elimination half-life 32–33 h), although elderly subjects are significantly impaired on psychomotor tests up to 36 h after an oral dose (Castleden *et al.* 1977). In sick elderly patients the elimination half-life is increased, due to a larger volume of distribution. In these patients it takes twice as long as in young subjects to reach steady-state plasma concentrations, but the actual levels and the total clearance time are the same (Iisalo *et al.* 1977; Kangas *et al.* 1979). This suggests that increased receptor sensitivity is the main reason for the altered response to nitrazepam in old age.

Withdrawal effects

Difficulty in withdrawing a hypnotic is the main reason for continued prescriptions. Dependence is a common problem with the barbiturates, but it is now recognized that prolonged use of the benzodiazepines may also cause dependence. Mild withdrawal symptoms include: anxiety, insomnia, dizziness, and headaches, and in severe cases there may be nausea, vomiting, tremors, postural hypotension and confusional, or paranoid psychoses (Anonymous 1979). This is mainly a problem with the long-acting benzodiazepines, but has also been reported with lorazepam (Howe 1980) and temazepam (Ratna 1981). It has been recommended that to minimize withdrawal symptoms, doses should be within the therapeutic range, short courses should be prescribed and withdrawal should be gradual (Committee on the Review of Medicines 1980).

It has been said that short- and intermediate-acting hypnotics may cause severe worsening of insomnia on withdawal (Kales *et al.* 1979), but a critical review concluded that there was little or no evidence that short acting hypnotics caused rebound insomnia (Nicholson 1980).

THE IDEAL HYPNOTIC

Such a drug would act rapidly to produce normal sleep, leave the patient refreshed and without hangover in the morning, and be non-addictive. Generally speaking the closest that one can get to this ideal is by using drugs with short elimination half-lives. Chlormethiazole, even in the elderly, has an elimination half-life of about 4 h with no evidence of accumulation after repeated doses (Briggs *et al.* 1980; Exton-Smith and Witts 1980). It is safe and effective in the elderly and does not cause significant hangover (Nayal *et al.* 1978). The usual dose is two capsules (384 mg of chlormethiazole base) or 10 ml of syrup and in these recommended doses it is relatively safe, the commonest side-effect being nasal irritation. Caution is necessary in chronic alcoholics and in patients with cirrhosis of the liver, because it is extensively metabolized in the liver.

Chloral hydrate and triclofos both produce the active metabolite trichloroethanol which has a plasma half-life of about 8 h. Triclofos is more pleasant to take and is an acceptable hypnotic for the elderly (Caplan *et al.* 1964). The usual dose is 1.5 g, but effectiveness declines after the first three nights (Kales *et al.* 1970) although side-effects are uncommon. Hangover, confusion, skin rashes, ataxia, and addiction may occur.

Temazepam, although relatively short-acting in young subjects, has a longer elimination half-life of 22 h in the elderly. It is an effective hypnotic (Briggs *et al.* 1980) but because of accumulation, adverse effects are seen with prolonged use (Cook 1980). Triazolam is said to have a very short elimination half-life of 2-3 h. In a dose of 0.125 mg it is free of hangover effects (Lipani 1978) and at present this is probably the benzodiazepine of choice for the elderly.

There are two situations where none of these hypnotics is the drug of choice. The first is the depressed patient with insomnia when a sedative antidepressant such as dothiepin may be given in a single 75 mg dose at bedtime. The second is the confused, agitated, restless patient who often responds best to thioridazine (50-100 mg) or haloperidol (1-5 mg).

Hypnotics to be avoided

Long-acting benzodiazepines can cause hangover effects in young subjects, but the risk of adverse reactions increases with age. Thus hangover following nitrazepam occurs in 0.9 per cent of those aged less than 40 years, rising to 4.4 per cent in those aged 70 or over, and 11.1 per cent in those over 80 years (Greenblatt and Allen 1978). A similar pattern has been reported with diazepam, chlordiazepoxide (Boston Collaborative Drug Surveillance Program 1973), and flurazepam (Greenblatt *et al.* 1977). These adverse reactions are cumulative and with flurazepam, for example, are most marked after three weeks of drug administration (Oswald 1979). These benzodiazepines should be avoided in the very old and the frail, and if used at all, given in the lowest doses, say nitrazepam 2.5 mg and flurazepam 15 mg. The hypnotic effect is not increased with larger doses.

Barbiturates are now contraindicated in the elderly except in special circumstances (Committee on the Review of Medicines 1979) and because of toxicity and the risk of abuse, glutethemide and methaqualone are also generally unsuitable.

CONCLUSIONS

Hypnotics should be prescribed only after careful evaluation of the patient, and then for a very limited period, say 10 days. The patient should be given a short-acting drug such as chlormethiazole or triazolam, and advised to take it only if he is still awake an hour after going to bed. Daytime naps and evening drinks of tea or coffee should be discouraged. Often the most effective cure for insomnia, but difficult to achieve, is for the person to increase his level of daytime activity. Social centres and day hospitals may be helpful.

REFERENCES

Anonymous (1979). Benzodiazepine withdrawal. *Lancet* i, 196.
Boston Collaborative Drug Surveillance Program (1973). Clinical depression of the central nervous system due to diazepam and chlordiazepoxide in relation to cigarette smoking and age. *New Engl. J. Med.* **288**, 277–80.
Breimer, D. D., Bracht, H., and de Boer, A. G. (1977). Plasma level profile of nitrazepam (Mogadon) following oral administration. *Br. J. clin. Pharmac.* **4**, 709–11.
Briggs, R. S., Castleden, C. M., and Kraft, C. A. (1980). Improved hypnotic treatment using chlormethiazole and temazepam. *Br. med. J.* **280**, 601–4.

Brocklehurst, J.C., Exton-Smith, A.N., Lempert Barber, S.M., and Palmer, M.K. (1977). Barbiturates and fractures. *Br. med. J.* ii, 699.
Caplan, H., Exton-Smith, A. N., and Hodkinson, H. M. (1964). Triclofos as a hypnotic in the elderly. *Practitioner* 192, 122–3.
Castleden, C. M., George, C. F., Marcer, D., and Hallett, C. (1977). Increased sensitivity to nitrazepam in old age. *Br. med. J.* i, 10–12.
Clift, A. D. (1972). Factors leading to dependence on hypnotic drugs. *Br. med. J.* iii, 614–17.
Committee on the Review of Medicines (1979). Recommendations on barbiturate preparations. *Br. med. J.* ii, 719–20.
— (1980). Systematic review of the benzodiazepines. *Br. med. J.* 280, 910–12.
Cook, P. (1980). Change in benzodiazepine drug activity with ageing. In *Current trends in therapeutics in the elderly* (ed. A. N. Exton-Smith). Medical Education (Services), Oxford.
Costello, C. G. and Smith, C. M. (1963). The relationship between personality, sleep and the effects of sedatives. *Br. J. Psychiat.* 109, 568–71.
Curry, S. H. and Whelpton, R. (1979). Pharmacokinetics of closely related benzodiazepines. *Br. J. clin. Pharmac.* 8, Suppl. 15S–21S.
Evans, J. G. and Jarvis, E. H. (1972). Nitrazepam and the elderly. *Br. med. J.* iv, 487.
Exton-Smith, A. N. and Witts, D. J. (1980). A comparison of chlormethiazole and nitrazepam as hypnotics in elderly subjects – with a note on the pharmacokinetics of chlormethiazole. In *Current trends in therapeutics in the elderly* (ed. A. N. Exton-Smith). Medical Education (Services), Oxford.
Fuccella, L. M. (1979). Bioavailability of temazepam in soft gelatin capsules. *Br. J. clin. Pharmac.* 8, 31S–5S.
Gerard, P., Collins, K. J., Dore, C., and Exton-Smith, A. N. (1978). Subjective characteristics of sleep in the elderly. *Age Ageing* 7, Suppl., 55–9.
Gibson, I. I. J. M. (1966). Barbiturate delirium. *Practitioner* 197, 345–7.
Greenblatt, D. J. and Allen, M. D. (1978). Toxicity of nitrazepam in the elderly. *Br. J. clin. Pharmac.* 5, 407–13.
— — and Shader, R.I. (1977). Toxicity of high dose flurazepam in the elderly. *Clin. Pharmac. Ther.* 21, 355–61.
Howe, J. G. (1980). Lorazepam withdrawal seizures. *Br. med. J.* 280, 1163–4.
Howell, T. H. (1960). Sedation and analgesia in old age. *Practitioner* 184, 45–8.
Iisalo, E., Kangas, L., and Ruikka, I. (1977). Pharmacokinetics of nitrazepam in young volunteers and aged patients. *Br. J. clin. Pharmac.* 4, 646P–7P.
Kales, A., Allen, C., Scharf, M. B., and Kales, J. D. (1970). Hypnotic drugs and their effectiveness. All-night e.e.g. studies of insomniac subjects. *Archs gen. Psychiat.* 23, 226–32.
— Bixler, E. O., Tan, T. L., Scharf, M. B., and Kales, J. D. (1974). Chronic hypnotic-drug use: ineffectiveness, drug-withdrawal insomnia and dependence. *J. Am. med. Ass.* 227, 513–17.
— and Kales, J. D. (1975). Shortcomings in the evaluation and promotion of hypnotic drugs. *New Engl. J. Med.* 293, 826–7.
— Scharf, M. B., Kales, J. D., and Soldatos, C. R. (1979). Rebound insomnia – a potential hazard following withdrawal of certain benzodiazepines. *J. Am. Med. Ass.* 241, 1692–5.
Kangas, L., Iisalo, E., Kanto, J., Lehtinen, V., Pynnönen, S., Ruikka, I. *et al.* (1979). Human pharmacokinetics in nitrazepam: effect of age and disease. *Eur. J. clin. Pharmac.* 15, 163–70.
Lipani, J. A. (1978). Preference study of the hypnotic efficacy of triazolam 0.125 mg compared to placebo in geriatric patients with insomnia. *Curr. Ther. Res.* 24, 397–402.
Macdonald, J. B. and Macdonald, E. T. (1977). Nocturnal femoral fracture and

continuing widespread use of barbiturate hypnotics. *Br. med. J.* ii, 483–5.
McGhie, A. and Russell, S. M. (1962). The subjective assessment of normal sleep patterns. *J. ment. Sci.* 108, 642–54.
Mendelson, W. B. (1980). *The use and misuse of sleeping pills.* Plenum Press, New York.
Nayal, S., Castleden, C. M., George, C. F., and Marcer, D. (1978). The effect of an hypnotic with a short half-life on hangover effect in old patients. *Age Ageing* 7, Suppl. 50–4.
Nicholson, A. N. (1980). Hypnotics: rebound insomnia and residual sequelae. *Br. J. clin. Pharmac.* 9, 223–5.
Oswald, I. (1979). The why and how of hypnotic drugs. *Br. med. J.* i, 1167–8.
— Březinová, V., and Carruthers-Jones, I. (1975). Sleep disorders to-day. In *Advanced medicine symposium II* (ed. A. F. Lant). Pitman Medical, Tunbridge Wells.
Ratna, L. (1981). Addiction to temazepam. *Br. med. J.* 282, 1837–8.
Rudd, T. N. (1972). Prescribing methods and iatrogenic situations in old age. *Geront. Clin.* 14, 123–8.
Wagner, J. G. (1967). Drug accumulation. *J. clin. Ph.. ..iac.* 7, 84–8.
Williams, R. L., Karacan, I., and Hursch, C. J. (1974). *Electroencephalography (EEG) of human sleep: clinical applications.* Wiley, New York.

15

Paranoid psychosis in the elderly

BRICE PITT

According to the *Oxford English Dictionary*, the literal meaning of the Greek word paranoia is 'beside the mind' (or 'beside oneself'), i.e. mentally deranged.

A useful review by Bridge and Wyatt (1980) points out that the term was introduced into the medical literature of the nineteenth century by Heinroth (1818), while Esquirol (1845) first used it in its current persecutory sense, when he discussed 'monomania intellectuelle'. Griesinger (1867) confirmed his view of the primacy of the delusions of the paranoid process, regarding paranoia as a disturbance of perception, intellect and thinking, with no understandable relationship to the patient's life.

PARAPHRENIA

Kraepelin (1919) devised the term *paraphrenia* for a state characterized by paranoia and hallucinations, and distinguished from dementia praecox by its late onset in life and failure to progress to personality disintegration. Since then there have been arguments about whether paraphrenia is an entity and to what extent it is distinguishable from schizophrenia (Kolle 1931; Mayer Gross 1932; Bleuler 1943). The term fell temporarily out of favour, until it was revived by Martin Roth (1955) who used it to describe a functional psychosis of late life, accounting for as many as 10 per cent of all elderly first admission patients. The condition comprized a well-organized system of paranoid delusions, with or without auditory hallucinations, existing in the setting of a well-preserved personality and affective response; that is to say, it was not secondary to confusion or a severe disturbance of mood. Despite a rearguard action by Fish (1960) who felt that there was no difference between so called paraphrenia and paranoid schizophrenia, the term has been perpetuated in Europe at least; in the United States, according to Bridge and Wyatt (1980), it is less familiar. But British psychogeriatricians, notably Post (1966), find that it designates a specific clinical disorder, in some ways resembling schizophrenia but arising much later in life (generally after the age of 60), being distinct from other mental illnesses of old age and remaining remarkably true to itself. It is hard not to concur with Post's (1978) view that the question of whether such patients are schizophrenics or paraphrenics is really meaningless; the writer's mildly irreverent but not wholly facetious concept of paraphrenia is as a sort of elderly aunt of schizophrenia. This at least indicates the genetic link between the two disorders, the characteristically schizophrenic nature of such manifestations of paraphrenia such as thought disorder and passivity feelings, and the special susceptibility of women.

While this chapter is mainly concerned with paraphrenia, it must be stated that a state of suspicion in the elderly is not always morbid, and that there are other causes for morbid suspicion than paraphrenia. Old people living alone and/or in a state of reluctant dependence because of physical infirmity, may well be *justified* in their fears that there are those who would take drastic decisions affecting them, without seeking their opinion or even informing them (e.g. over transfer to continuing care from an acute ward); or who would exploit their weakness by robbing and assaulting them. Agism (Butler 1975) is very prevalent in societies where there are large numbers of the elderly, and old people are easy victims for confidence tricksters and muggers. It might well behove many of the elderly to be less trusting and gullible and more suspicious.

Then paranoid states in the elderly may be *secondary* to confusion, depression or mania, or may arise from a paranoid personality in conflict with those with whom the sufferer has contact. The paranoia of the *delirious* is fleeting and fluctuates, generally according to the degree of clouding of consciousness. The paranoid phase of *dementia* usually involves no more than the belief that things mislaid have been stolen, or a catastrophic reaction of noisy indignation when the limitations of intellect and memory are threatened with exposure. Some severely *depressed* old people believe that others share their low opinion of themselves and talk about it, while the *manic* elderly may feel paranoid towards those who would thwart them. Paranoid *personalities* are very likely to be quite alone in old age, and if they then become infirm and need help they are far from mellow and appreciative, but querulous, accusatory, and much inclined to 'bite the hand which feeds them'. The distinction between these disorders and paraphrenia is generally clear, but difficulty sometimes arises (see below).

Certain conditions are said to *predispose* to paranoia, whether arising in the context of paraphrenia or other paranoid states, and include the circumstances now to be described.

Sensory deprivation

Deafness is one of the most important manifestations in this context, as has been emphasized in Chapter 11. Levine (1960) commented that 'while deafness does not itself produce mental illness, it does by its very nature provoke paranoid ideas in sensitive individuals, by keeping them from direct contact with what others in the environment are saying and thinking, thus laying the foundation for suspicion'. Cooper *et al.* (1974, 1976) compared elderly patients with paraphrenia and with affective illness, matched for age and sex, and concluded that the paraphrenic had hearing losses of significantly greater magnitude and duration than did the affectively ill. (Thomas (1981) has, however, pointed out that studies which look for paranoia among the deaf, rather than deafness among the paranoid, are less persuasive.) Deaf old people are certainly liable to be treated with as much exasperation as sympathy, and to be talked about rather than to.

The *blind* are more likely to be regarded with compassion, but the acute loss of sight which follows some ophthalmic surgery, though usually only temporary, until the bandages are removed, is sometimes associated with a transitory paranoid reaction. Cooper and Porter (1976) found that paraphrenics had significantly more cataracts and more far vision problems in the worse eye, than elderly affectively ill patients.

Any major hospital procedure which leaves the patient apprehensive, baffled, uninformed, uncomfortable, and unable to move much, e.g. intensive care, may precipitate acute paranoia.

Social factors

Debility and *exhaustion*, such as may be wilfully induced by brain washing or arise from chronic painful illness, readily induce a peevish, self-pitying sensitivity. Occasionally, when an invalid feels neglected or discriminated against, this becomes frankly paranoid.

A *foreign* environment has already been implicated in Chapter 12. Immigrants are notoriously liable to paranoid reactions, ranging from the very common fears of prejudice and victimization, to florid illness. For many old people, hospitals and homes are a foreign environment, and often many of the staff are foreign.

Illiteracy is conducive to paranoia, because it is not only an obstacle to obtaining information but a source of shame.

Physical factors

Drugs, such as steroids, L-dopa, benzhexol, and (though rarely in the elderly) amphetamines, in excessive quantities may provoke paranoid reactions. Chronic alcoholism is significantly associated with paranoid psychosis.

Certain *physical diseases* affecting the brain without causing delirium or dementia, can cause paranoia, which is one form of Asher's (1949) 'myxoedematous madness', and tends to develop in severe epileptics after several years of their illness.

DIAGNOSTIC FEATURES

Returning to the specific topic of *paraphrenia*, the typical patient is, according to Kay and Roth's study (1961), female, solitary, partially deaf, and eccentric, but without a past history of psychiatric illness. In this respect there is a marked difference from the elderly depressive. In later life, usually in the senium, she starts to build up suspicions of her neighbours and believes that they comment on and criticize her. This belief may be based on ideas of reference or auditory hallucinations — voices which talk about her disparagingly, abuse or instruct her, and which she generally hears only at home, but which may pursue her wherever she goes. She may well believe that she is spied upon with telescopes or television cameras, with wireless, microphones, and tape recorders; that noxious gases are blown in, strange lights are shone (though visual phenomena are rarely prominent), that powder is sprinkled on her food, the water poisoned, that she is attacked with radiation, and that her electricity is stolen. Often there is thought to be a mysterious machine, operating night and day, which keeps the patient awake though no one else can hear it.

Erotic delusions are not unknown, with passivity feelings of rape from afar, and a poignant variation is that a child nearby is being ill treated (Pitt 1982). The delusions are usually strictly localized and well sustained. The response to them is usually appropriate, i.e. to be distressed, seek rehousing, complain to the police, retaliate or go into a state of siege. Sometimes metonyms and neologisms are used to describe the weird goings on, though thought disorder is never more extensive.

Both Kay and Roth (1961) and Post (1966) have proposed that there are three variations of paraphrenia. The Newcastle workers suggested different aetiologies:

(a) abnormal personalities with paranoia but no hallucinations;
(b) arising under unusual circumstances, or after prolonged isolation;
(c) 'endogenous' paranoia.

Post describes paranoid, schizophreniform and schizophrenic subgroups:

(i) paranoid delusions and hallucinations are strictly localized;
(ii) more widespread delusions spread into the neighbourhood and the street, notions of being spied upon are more complex and elaborate, and there may be jealous delusions about the spouse;
(iii) the picture is virtually that of paranoid schizophrenia, with passivity feelings, some thought disorder and voices discussing the patient in the third person.

Post does not claim that these forms of paraphrenia differ in aetiology, or in response to treatment, but they tend to stay true to type.

Prevalence

In a comprehensive psychogeriatric service, taking all psychiatric referrals from the population aged 65 and over in a defined catchment area, 9 per cent were diagnosed at first assessment as having a paranoid state; the great majority were later diagnosed specifically as suffering from paraphrenia. All cases found in the Kay *et al.* (1964) survey of Newcastle upon Tyne, were found in hospital or homes; there were none among the 208 people aged over 65 and living at home. However, Williamson *et al.* (1964) found paranoid states in two women among 200 people over 65 at home in Edinburgh, and Parsons (1965) four out of 228 in Swansea, so the prevalence may be about 1 per cent, i.e. similar to that of schizophrenia. It seems that cases of paraphrenia may be better known than those of the other psychiatric disorders of old age, presumably because of the disruption they are liable to cause.

Aetiology

Five factors are involved, the first being the *genetic* one. The risk of schizophrenia among the close relatives of paraphrenics is greater than that of the general population, but less than that of younger schizophrenics. There is an expectancy rate for schizophrenia of 2.5 per cent among the siblings of paraphrenics, compared with 0.9 per cent in the population at large and 7.4 per cent in younger schizophrenics (Funding 1961). Kay and Roth (1961) not only found a 3.4 per cent incidence of schizophrenia kin for their paraphrenic patients, but eight paraphrenic siblings of their 99 probands. The striking excess of female over male patients also suggests a genetic factor (Post 1978).

The next factor involves *personality*. Although generally having a good work record, no tendency to show social decline and much less previous psychiatric illness than affectively ill older patients (Kay *et al.* 1976), paraphrenics have usually been withdrawn, with a poor capacity for close relationships, and a a tendency to eccentricity. They are often recluses at the onset of the psychosis.

Marital status is important and in a Stockholm group, Kay (1963) found that over a quarter of paraphrenics had had illegitimate children and that they rarely married the father. If they married at all, they tended to do so late.

Physical factors have already been mentioned. Paraphrenics tend to be physically healthier than elderly depressives, but more liable to deafness (Cooper *et al.* 1974; and see above). Post (1966) found that 15 per cent of his paraphrenics became demented over the course of three years observation, and dementia could not be ruled out in another 18 per cent; it is questionable, though, that the first figure would not apply to any group of like age followed over the same time.

Psychological factors also play a part. Sjogren (1964) felt that such aspects of aging as being in a disadvantaged group, isolation and loneliness, as well as faulty perception, and misinterpretation, contributed to paraphrenia. Retterstöl (1968) emphasized the reactive element, regarding psychological trauma as often causative. A quarter of Kay and Roth's (1961) cases were related to traumatic events (rather less than in those who became affectively ill). The writer has seen two cases of paraphrenic '*folie a deux*' in his psychogeriatric practice in the last year; one in a woman dutifully looking after here paraphrenic elderly sister, another in a man of rather low intelligence, seemingly eagerly seizing upon and reinforcing the delusions of his dominated, primarily paraphrenic wife.

Post (1978) puts the general view of British workers that the abnormal previous personalities of paraphrenic patients might be evidence of a longstanding latent schizophrenic disorder, which is finally brought into the open by the further social deprivations of late life, by deafness and by some cerebral aspects of the aging process.

Differential diagnosis

When paranoia is secondary to confusion, the history (if obtainable) should indicate that the confusion came first, while mental state should exhibit significant loss of recent memory. When depression is primary, there may well be a previous and family history of affective illness, depression should have preceded the paranoia and should be very evident at examination. Paranoid personalities have long been so, and their paranoia is more consistent with a jaundiced, cynical, misanthropic outlook than with a delusional system. Difficulties of differentiation arise, however, when the confused patient holds quite elaborate, florid, and bizarre delusions (though they tend to be poorly systematized) or when the extent and duration of a depressive's paranoia goes beyond what is readily explained by the severity of the effective disturbance. For example, an elderly married woman admitted with depression, delusions of poverty and unworthiness, and suicidal thoughts, became frankly hostile in hospital, believing that she was being misrepresented, slandered, and poisoned. A widow who had had to repay the Social Security money to which her late husband had not been entitled, had troublesome ideas of reference, long after her depression had apparently begun to lift. Of course, dementia and depressive illness are much the commonest psychiatric illnesses of late life, and must occasionally coincide with paraphrenia and not necessarily be its cause or consequence.

TREATMENT

Lacking insight, the paraphrenic is unlikely to seek medical aid except to relieve sleeplessness and general distress secondary to the feeling of being persecuted, or unless the doctor is seen as a powerful potential ally against the persecutors. Instead the police are often approached and, by a tactful, good humoured response, may well be able to support some of the milder cases. Rehousing is often sought and obtained, and may be temporarily beneficial except to the more overtly schizophrenic, but the persecution is usually resumed within weeks or months. Other social measures such as befriending or arranging attendance at a club, day centre or hospital, may well help the patient to live with her delusions and reduce their intensity, but are inapplicable to most paraphrenics because of their lack of sociability.

Neuroleptic drugs

There is no doubt (Post 1966) that the potentially most effective treatment is with *phenothiazines*, but there are major problems of compliance. It is fruitless to argue with the patient about her delusions. Often, without agreeing whole-heartedly, one goes along with them or, at best, agrees to differ. Treatment may then be rationalized as a means of fortifying the patient against her harrassment, or while accepting the remote possibility that there could be substance in the patient's complaints, explaining that they are far more likely to arise from mental illness, and suggesting clarification by a trial of medication. Not infrequently, as Post has pointed out, the patient's attitude is ambivalent and if there is reasonable rapport with the prescriber, treatment is accepted even though it is inconsistent with the delusional beliefs. Sometimes a trusted general practitioner is more likely to achieve the rapport needed than a strange psychiatrist.

Some patients, then, can be treated with oral medication at home. Attendance at an outpatient clinic or day hospital or visits from a community psychogeriatric nurse, improve compliance and supervision. Compliance may be further improved by the use of depot injections in some cases. Compulsory admission may occasionally be justified, as for example when the patient is experiencing or causing extreme distress, especially as the results of treatment are likely to be good.

Because of the risk of side-effects (mainly extrapyramidal) oral medication is preferable to intramuscular, and the blander to the more neuroleptic drugs. Thus, if compliance seems likely, thioridazine is the preparation of first choice, in divided doses which may be increased to a total of 300 mg daily. If that fails, trifluoperazine would be tried next, in doses from 10 to 45 mg per day, given either in divided dosage as 5 mg tablets, or, preferably, once daily in 10–15 mg slow release spansules. Haloperidol has the questionable advantage that it may be presented in a colourless liquid (0.1 mg per drop) which may be discreetly incorporated in the patient's diet, at home if there is someone to, say, stir it into the tea, or in hospital. The dosage (divided) is up to 6 mg per day. This technique, which in a way realizes some of the patient's paranoid fears, is more expedient than ethical.

If an injection proves necessary it is wise to start with a test dose of fluphenazine enanthate 6.25 mg or flupenthixol 10 mg and observe the effects over the next week or two. Most patients will be adequately maintained on 25 mg of the former or 20 mg of the latter monthly, but occasionally it is necessary to give twice the dose twice as often.

Usually hallucinations dwindle away within two or three weeks of commencing treatment and delusions become far less troublesome, though full insight is rarely obtained. The chief side-effects of medication are drowsiness (because of sedation), dizziness (due to hypotension), and extrapyramidal effects: tremor, stiffness, ataxia, akathesia, and drooling. There is also a distinct risk of tardive dyskynesia, which may be increased by the routine use of anti-Parkinsonian drugs, which should therefore be withheld unless there are signs that they are needed; orphenadrine, 150–300 mg daily in divided dosage may then be given. Depression occasionally develops in the course of treatment and may require antidepressants.

Precautions

It was disconcerting to find that the commonest iatrogenic cause of admissions to a joint geriatric/psychogeriatric unit (Pitt and Silver 1980) was the use of depot phenothiazine injections. The following precautions should therefore be observed:

(i) treat only when the disorder is truly troublesome;
(ii) be especially cautious in the presence of confusion or physical infirmity;
(iii) use the lowest possible effective dose;
(iv) use oral medication wherever compliance seems likely;
(v) use anti-Parkinsonian drugs at the first sign of side-effects;
(vi) reduce the dosage as soon as possible, try 'drug holidays';
(vii) maintain close supervision.

Post (1966) found that of 71 paraphrenics treated with oral medication, 14 (20 per cent) recovered fully, 29 (42 per cent) recovered fully without full insight, 22 (31 per cent) made social recoveries only retaining some abnormal ideas, and only six (8 per cent) made no improvement at all.

Prognosis

Over an average follow up period of three years in Post's study, prognosis was closely related to the maintenance of drug therapy. Three-quarters of those making a full recovery remained well, but it was possible to stop the drugs lastingly in only 16 per cent of these. Other good prognostic features than continuing compliance were:

(a) immediate response to treatment;
(b) the development of insight;
(c) marriage;
(d) relative youth.

Untreated, paraphrenia tends to pursue a chronic unremitting course, and once fully developed is likely to continue unchanged until the patient's death.

Life expectancy, however, is at least that of the elderly population at large, with a lower mortality rate than that of the demented or affectively ill (Kay and Roth 1961).

CONCLUSIONS

Many old people are rightly suspicious, but a morbid state of suspicion is, after depression and confusion, the commonest presentation of psychiatric disorder in old age, accounting for about 10 per cent of referrals. The basis may be confusion, affective disorder, or a paranoid personality; but is most often paraphrenia, a primary schizophreniform psychosis characterized by its late onset in life, strongly held systematized and localized paranoid delusions (and, often, auditory hallucinations), and the absence of personality deterioration. The family history of paraphrenia and schizophrenia exceeds that of the general population but, of the latter, is less than that of younger schizophrenics. The disorder predominates in women of a solitary and somewhat eccentric nature, living alone and partially deaf. A past history of mental illness and precipitation by life events are less common than in affectively ill older patients. Social measures are of some small value. Phenothiazines are effective in the treatment of paraphrenia, but compliance and side-effects are problems. Prognosis is closely linked to the maintenance of therapy, but whether treated or not, paraphrenia does not reduce life expectancy.

Acknowledgement

I should like to express my appreciation to Dr Peter Grahame for his help in the preparation of this chapter.

REFERENCES

Asher, R. (1949). Myxoedematous madness. *Br. med. J.* ii, 555.
Bleuler, M. (1943). Die spaet schizophrenen Krankhiltsbilden. *Fortsch. Neurol. Psychiat.* 15, 259.
Bridge, T. P. and Wyatt, R. O. (1980). Paraphrenia: paranoid states of late life. I European research. *J. Am. geriat. Soc.* 28, 193.
—— —— (1980). Paraphrenia: paranoid states of late life. II American research. *J. Am. geriat. Soc.* 28, 201.
Butler, R. N. (1975). *Why survive? Being old in America.* Harper and Row, New York.
Cooper, A. F., Curry, A. R., Kay, D. W. K., Garside, R. F., and Roth, M. (1974). Hearing loss in paranoid and affective psychoses of the elderly. *Lancet* ii, 851.
—— Garside, R.F., and Kay, D.W.K. (1976). A comparison of deaf and non-deaf patients with paranoid and affective psychoses. *Br. J. Psychiat.* 129, 297.
—— and Porter, R. (1976). Visual acuity and ocular pathology in the paranoid and affective psychoses of late life. *J. psychosomat. Res.* 20, 107.
Esquirol, E. (1845). *Mental maladies* (transl. E. K. Hunt). Lee and Blanchard, Philadelphia.
Fish, F. (1960). Senile schizophrenia. *J. ment. Sci.* 106, 938.
Funding, T. (1961). Genetics of paranoid psychoses of later life. *Acta psychiat. scand.* 37, 267.
Griesinger, W. (1867). *Mental pathology and therapeutics* (trans. C.L. Robertson and L. Rutherford). New Sydenham Society, London.

Heinroth, J. C. A. (1825). *System der Psychisch Gerichtlichen Medicin*. Hartman, Leipzig.

Kay, D. W. K. (1963). Late paraphrenia and its bearing on the aetiology of schizophrenia. *Acta psychiat. scand.* **39**, 159.

— Beamish, P., and Roth, M. (1964). Old age mental disorders in Newcastle upon Tyne. I: Prevalence. *Br. J. Psychiat.* **110**, 146.

— Cooper, A., Garside, R. F., and Roth, M. (1976). The differentiation of paranoid from affective psychoses by patients' premorbid characteristics. *Br. J. Psychiat.* **129**, 207;

— and Roth, M. (1961). Environmental and hereditary factors in the schizophrenias of old age ('late paraphrenia') and their bearing on the general problem of causation in schizophrenia. *J. ment. Sci.* **107**, 649.

Kolle, K. (1931). *Die Primare Verrucktheit*. Thieme, Leipzig.

Kraepelin, E. (1919). *Dementia pracox and paraphrenia*. Krieger, New York.

Levine, E. D. (1960). *The psychology of deafness: techniques of appraisal for rehabilitation*. Columbia University Press, New York.

Mayer Gross, W. (1932). *Die Schizophrenie*. Springer, Berlin.

Parsons, P. (1965). Mental health of Swansea's old folk. *Br. J. prevent. soc. Med.* **19**, 43.

Pitt, B. (1982). *Psychogeriatrics*, 2nd edn. Churchill Livingstone, Edinburgh.

— and Silver, C.P. (1980). The combined approach to geriatrics and psychiatry: evaluation of a joint unit in a teaching hospital district. *Age Ageing* **9**, 33.

Post, F. (1966). *Persistent persecutory states of the elderly*. Pergamon Press, Oxford.

— (1978). The functional psychoses. In *Studies in geriatric psychiatry* (ed. A. D. Isaacs and F. Post). Wiley, Chichester.

Retterstöl, N. (1968). Paranoid psychoses. *Br. J. Psychiat.* **114**, 533.

Roth, M. (1955). The natural history of mental disorder in old age. *J. ment. Sci.* **101**, 281.

Sjogren, H. (1964). Paraphrenic, melancholic and psychoneurotic states in the presenile/senile period of life. *Acta psychiat. scand.* Suppl., 176.

Thomas, A. J. (1981). Acquired deafness and mental health. *Br. J. med. Psychol.* **54**, 219.

Williamson, J., Stokoe, I., Gray, S., Fisher, M., Smith, A., McGhee, A., and Stephenson, E. (1964). Old people at home: their unreported needs. *Lancet* **i**, 1117.

Index